Empowering Kids: A Comprehensive Guide to Managing Anxiety

Table of Contents:

Chapter 1: Understanding Anxiety in Kids
- 1.1 What is Anxiety?
  - 1.1.1 Types of Anxiety Disorders
- 1.2 Recognizing Anxiety in Children
  - 1.2.1 Common Signs and Symptoms
  - 1.2.2 Triggers and Causes

Chapter 2: The Importance of Early Intervention
- 2.1 The Impact of Childhood Anxiety
  - 2.1.1 Academic Performance
  - 2.1.2 Social Development
  - 2.1.3 Long-term Consequences
- 2.2 Seeking Professional Help
  - 2.2.1 Pediatricians and Child Psychologists
  - 2.2.2 Therapeutic Approaches

Chapter 3: Building a Supportive Environment
- 3.1 Open Communication
  - 3.1.1 Creating a Safe Space
  - 3.1.2 Active Listening
- 3.2 Setting Realistic Expectations
  - 3.2.1 Balancing Academics and Extracurriculars
  - 3.2.2 Encouraging Self-Care

Chapter 4: Coping Strategies for Kids
- 4.1 Mindfulness and Relaxation Techniques
  - 4.1.1 Deep Breathing Exercises
  - 4.1.2 Guided Imagery
- 4.2 Cognitive Behavioral Techniques
  - 4.2.1 Identifying Negative Thoughts
  - 4.2.2 Positive Self-Talk

Chapter 5: Healthy Lifestyle Habits
- 5.1 The Connection Between Diet and Anxiety
  - 5.1.1 Nutrient-Rich Foods
  - 5.1.2 Limiting Sugar and Caffeine
- 5.2 The Role of Exercise in Anxiety Management
  - 5.2.1 Fun Physical Activities for Kids
  - 5.2.2 The Power of Play

Chapter 6: Managing Anxiety at School
- 6.1 Talking to Teachers and School Counselors
  - 6.1.1 Individualized Education Plans (IEPs)
  - 6.1.2 Reducing Academic Pressure
- 6.2 Creating a Safe Space at School

- 6.2.1 Peer Support
- 6.2.2 Stress-Free Study Tips

Chapter 7: Nurturing Resilience and Self-esteem
- 7.1 Encouraging Problem-Solving Skills
  - 7.1.1 Facing Fears Gradually
  - 7.1.2 Learning from Mistakes
- 7.2 Building Self-confidence
  - 7.2.1 Celebrating Achievements
  - 7.2.2 Embracing Uniqueness

Chapter 8: Coping with Specific Anxiety Challenges
- 8.1 Separation Anxiety
  - 8.1.1 Transitioning Smoothly
  - 8.1.2 Building Trust
- 8.2 Test and Performance Anxiety
  - 8.2.1 Effective Study Techniques
  - 8.2.2 Relaxation Rituals

Chapter 9: Sibling and Family Dynamics
- 9.1 The Impact of Anxiety on Family
  - 9.1.1 Empathy and Understanding
  - 9.1.2 Sibling Support
- 9.2 Family Bonding Activities
  - 9.2.1 Quality Time Together
  - 9.2.2 Group Problem-Solving

Chapter 10: Thriving Beyond Anxiety
- 10.1 Monitoring Progress
  - 10.1.1 Keeping a Journal
  - 10.1.2 Tracking Achievements
- 10.2 Celebrating Successes
  - 10.2.1 Gradual Steps Toward Independence
  - 10.2.2 Planning for the Future

Chapter 11: Resources for Parents and Caregivers
- 11.1 Books and Websites
- 11.2 Support Groups and Counseling Services
- 11.3 Advocacy and Awareness Organizations

Chapter 12: Conclusion
- 12.1 The Journey Ahead
- 12.2 Empowering Kids for Life

In "Empowering Kids: A Comprehensive Guide to Managing Anxiety," parents, caregivers, educators, and children will find valuable insights, practical strategies, and a holistic approach to help kids effectively cope with anxiety. From understanding the roots of anxiety to fostering resilience and self-esteem, this book provides a roadmap for nurturing happy, confident, and anxiety-resilient children.

Chapter 1: Understanding Anxiety in Kids

Introduction

Anxiety is a natural and common human emotion. It's a response that has evolved over thousands of years to help us deal with danger and uncertainty. In its essence, anxiety is the body's way of preparing for a potential threat. It's the reason our ancestors survived in a world filled with predators and unknown dangers. However, in today's modern world, anxiety can sometimes become excessive and overwhelming, especially for our children.

In this first chapter, we embark on a journey to understand anxiety in the context of children. We'll delve into the complex world of this emotion and explore how it manifests in the lives of our youngest generation. It's essential to remember that children, like adults, experience anxiety, but their understanding and coping mechanisms are still developing. As caregivers, parents, educators, and friends, it's our responsibility to recognize and support them through their anxiety struggles.

But before we explore strategies for helping children manage anxiety, we need to lay the foundation by answering some fundamental questions. What is anxiety, exactly? How does it differ in children compared to adults? What are the common signs and symptoms to look out for? And what are the potential triggers and causes that might be contributing to a child's anxiety?

As we navigate through this chapter, you'll gain a deeper understanding of the intricate nature of childhood anxiety. You'll learn to recognize its various manifestations and, most importantly, appreciate that anxiety is not something to be ashamed of or ignored. Instead, it's a challenge that can be addressed and managed, paving the way for a happier, more confident, and resilient future for the children in our lives.

So, let's embark on this enlightening journey together, as we unravel the mysteries of anxiety in kids and equip ourselves with the knowledge and empathy needed to provide the support and guidance that every child deserves.

1.1 What is Anxiety?

Anxiety is a natural and universal human emotion that all of us experience at various points in our lives. It's a complex emotional state characterized by feelings of unease, apprehension, or fear. Anxiety serves an evolutionary purpose, originating from our ancestors' need to stay alert in the face of potential dangers and threats. When properly regulated, anxiety can motivate us to take action and make prudent decisions.

In essence, anxiety can be thought of as our body's alarm system, designed to protect us from harm. When we encounter a situation perceived as threatening, whether it's a physical danger or a psychological stressor, our brain triggers a series of physiological responses. These responses include the release of stress hormones like cortisol and adrenaline, which prepare our bodies to respond quickly to the perceived threat. This "fight or flight" response can be life-saving in certain situations.

In children, anxiety plays a crucial role in their development. It can help them learn to navigate the world, assess risks, and develop problem-solving skills. However, when anxiety becomes chronic or excessive, it can interfere with a child's daily life and well-being.

It's important to note that anxiety exists on a spectrum. Some level of anxiety is entirely normal and can even be beneficial. However, when anxiety becomes overwhelming, persistent, or irrational, it may be classified as an anxiety disorder. Anxiety disorders encompass a range of conditions, such as generalized anxiety disorder (GAD), social anxiety disorder, panic disorder, and specific phobias, among others.

In the context of children, understanding the nuances of anxiety is crucial. They may not always have the language or self-awareness to express their feelings accurately. Therefore, caregivers and adults must be attuned to the signs and symptoms of anxiety in children, as well as the factors that can contribute to its development.

In the sections that follow, we'll explore how anxiety can manifest in children, the specific challenges they face, and how to differentiate normal childhood worries from more significant anxiety issues. By gaining a deeper understanding of anxiety in children, we can better support them on their journey to emotional well-being and resilience.

1.1.1 Types of Anxiety Disorders

Anxiety disorders encompass a diverse group of mental health conditions, each characterized by distinct patterns of excessive and debilitating anxiety. While anxiety itself is a normal and adaptive emotion, these disorders involve chronic and often irrational levels of fear and worry that interfere with daily life. In the context of children, it's essential to recognize the various types of anxiety disorders, as they can manifest differently in younger individuals. Here are some of the most common anxiety disorders affecting children:

1. Generalized Anxiety Disorder (GAD): Generalized Anxiety Disorder is marked by excessive worry and anxiety about a wide range of everyday concerns. Children with GAD may worry excessively about their academic performance, friendships, family issues, and various other aspects of their lives. This constant worry often leads to physical symptoms like restlessness, muscle tension, and difficulty concentrating.

2. Social Anxiety Disorder: Social anxiety disorder, also known as social phobia, is characterized by an intense fear of social situations and performance situations. Children with social anxiety may fear being embarrassed or humiliated in front of others, leading to avoidance of social interactions, public speaking, or participating in group activities.

3. Separation Anxiety Disorder: Separation anxiety disorder is common in younger children and involves extreme distress when separated from primary caregivers or familiar environments. Children with this disorder may exhibit clinginess, refusal to attend school or be left alone, nightmares about separation, and physical symptoms like stomachaches or headaches.

4. Specific Phobias: Specific phobias involve intense and irrational fears of particular objects or situations. Common childhood phobias include fear of animals, heights, thunderstorms, needles, and the dark. These fears can significantly disrupt a child's life if left unaddressed.

5. Panic Disorder: While less common in children than in adults, panic disorder can occur in childhood. It involves recurrent and unexpected panic attacks, which are intense episodes of extreme fear or discomfort accompanied by physical symptoms such as a rapid heartbeat, sweating, and shortness of breath. Children with panic disorder may also develop a fear of having future panic attacks.

6. Obsessive-Compulsive Disorder (OCD): OCD is characterized by the presence of obsessions (intrusive and distressing thoughts) and compulsions (repetitive behaviors or mental acts performed to reduce anxiety). Children with OCD may engage in rituals like excessive handwashing, checking, or counting to alleviate their obsessive thoughts.

7. Post-Traumatic Stress Disorder (PTSD): While typically associated with exposure to traumatic events, PTSD can affect children who have experienced or witnessed distressing events. Symptoms may include flashbacks, nightmares, avoidance of reminders, and heightened arousal.

Understanding these different types of anxiety disorders is a crucial first step in recognizing and addressing anxiety-related challenges in children. Each disorder presents its unique set of symptoms and requires tailored approaches to assessment, treatment, and support. In the chapters ahead, we'll explore how to identify these disorders and provide effective strategies for helping children manage their anxiety.

1.2 Recognizing Anxiety in Children

Recognizing anxiety in children can be both challenging and essential. Unlike adults, children may not always have the vocabulary or self-awareness to articulate their feelings accurately. Anxiety often manifests differently in younger individuals, and its signs can be subtle or easily mistaken for normal childhood behaviors. As caregivers, parents, and educators, it's crucial to be attentive and observant to identify anxiety in children effectively.

1.2.1 Common Signs and Symptoms

Understanding the common signs and symptoms of anxiety in children is a vital first step in recognizing their emotional struggles. Keep in mind that not all children will exhibit the same signs, and the intensity of symptoms can vary. Here are some common indicators of anxiety in children:

1. Excessive Worry: Children with anxiety may worry excessively about various aspects of their lives, such as school performance, friendships, family matters, or even future events. Their worries often exceed what is developmentally appropriate.

2. Physical Symptoms: Anxiety can manifest physically in children. They may complain of stomachaches, headaches, muscle tension, fatigue, or other physical discomforts without an underlying medical cause.

3. Avoidance Behavior: Children with anxiety may avoid situations, people, or places that trigger their anxiety. This could include avoiding school, refusing to sleep alone, or not participating in social activities.

4. Perfectionism: Some anxious children may display perfectionistic tendencies, setting unrealistically high standards for themselves and experiencing intense distress when they fail to meet them.

5. Restlessness: Anxiety can manifest as restlessness or an inability to sit still. Children may appear fidgety, have difficulty concentrating, or exhibit impulsive behavior.

6. Sleep Disturbances: Anxiety can disrupt a child's sleep patterns, leading to difficulties falling asleep,

frequent nightmares, or night sweats.

7. Irritability: Anxiety can make children irritable and easily upset. They may have outbursts of frustration or anger that seem disproportionate to the situation.

8. Social Withdrawal: Some anxious children may withdraw from social interactions, preferring solitude over spending time with peers.

9. Seek Reassurance: Anxious children often seek constant reassurance from parents or caregivers to alleviate their worries. They may repeatedly ask questions like, "Are you sure everything will be okay?" or "Do you still love me?"

1.2.2 Triggers and Causes

Understanding the triggers and potential causes of anxiety in children can provide valuable insights into their emotional struggles. Anxiety can result from a combination of genetic, environmental, and situational factors. Common triggers and causes of anxiety in children include:

1. Genetics: There may be a genetic predisposition to anxiety disorders, as they can run in families.

2. Environmental Stressors: Exposure to stressful family dynamics, financial difficulties, divorce, or other challenging life events can contribute to childhood anxiety.

3. Traumatic Events: Experiencing or witnessing traumatic events, such as accidents, natural disasters, or violence, can lead to post-traumatic stress and anxiety in children.

4. School Pressures: Academic pressures, bullying, or social challenges at school can trigger anxiety in children.

5. Parental Anxiety: Children may pick up on their parents' anxiety or coping styles, which can influence their own anxiety levels.

6. Major Life Transitions: Significant life changes, such as moving to a new school, a new home, or the arrival of a new sibling, can trigger anxiety in children.

By recognizing the signs and understanding potential triggers and causes, caregivers and educators can take proactive steps to support anxious children effectively. In the chapters ahead, we'll explore strategies for providing the necessary guidance and assistance to help children cope with anxiety and lead happier, more fulfilling lives.

Chapter 2: The Importance of Early Intervention

Introduction

Anxiety, whether in adults or children, is a powerful and pervasive force that can significantly impact one's quality of life. When it comes to our youngest generation, the effects of anxiety can be particularly profound, influencing their emotional well-being, social development, academic success, and overall happiness. Understanding the importance of early intervention in managing childhood anxiety is not only crucial but can be life-changing for a child's future.

In this chapter, we delve into the significance of recognizing and addressing anxiety in children as early as possible. Anxiety disorders in childhood are not merely a phase that children will eventually outgrow; they are real and treatable conditions that require attention and support. The impact of untreated childhood anxiety can be far-reaching, affecting various aspects of a child's life and potentially leading to long-term consequences.

We will explore how childhood anxiety can affect academic performance, social interactions, and emotional development. By gaining insight into the potential consequences of untreated anxiety, we can better appreciate the urgency of early intervention.

Early intervention involves seeking help and support for a child's anxiety challenges at the earliest signs or symptoms. This proactive approach aims to prevent the escalation of anxiety-related difficulties and provides children with the tools they need to navigate their emotions effectively.

As caregivers, parents, educators, and concerned individuals, we play a crucial role in recognizing when a child may be struggling with anxiety and taking the necessary steps to provide support. Through early intervention, we can empower children to manage their anxiety, develop resilience, and lead fulfilling lives unburdened by the weight of excessive worry and fear.

Join us on this journey as we explore the significance of early intervention in addressing childhood anxiety and discover practical strategies to identify, understand, and assist children who may be grappling with this complex emotion. Together, we can ensure that every child receives the help they need to thrive emotionally, socially, and academically.

2.1 The Impact of Childhood Anxiety

Childhood is a time of wonder, exploration, and growth. It's a period when children should be free to discover their interests, build friendships, and develop essential life skills. However, when anxiety enters the picture, it can cast a shadow over these formative years, profoundly influencing a child's life in various ways. In this section, we explore the far-reaching impact of childhood anxiety on a child's emotional well-being, social development, and academic success.

2.1.1 Academic Performance

One of the most noticeable and immediate areas where childhood anxiety can have a significant impact is in the realm of academics. Anxiety can affect a child's ability to focus, concentrate, and learn effectively. Here's how anxiety can manifest in relation to school:

- Impaired Concentration: Anxious children often struggle to concentrate on tasks, leading to difficulty completing assignments or following classroom instructions.

- Test and Performance Anxiety: Anxiety can trigger extreme stress before exams or when required to perform in front of others. This can hinder a child's ability to showcase their true capabilities.

- School Avoidance: In severe cases, some children may develop school avoidance behaviors due to their anxiety. They may refuse to attend school, which can lead to educational setbacks.

- Perfectionism: Anxiety can fuel perfectionistic tendencies in some children, making them fear mistakes and imperfections. This fear can paralyze their ability to take risks and engage in learning experiences.

2.1.2 Social Development

Childhood is a critical period for the development of social skills, relationships, and a sense of belonging. Anxiety can profoundly impact a child's social development:

- Social Isolation: Anxious children may withdraw from social interactions, leading to feelings of loneliness and isolation. This isolation can hinder their ability to develop close friendships and healthy social connections.

- Peer Rejection: Anxiety-related behaviors, such as excessive shyness or fearfulness, can sometimes lead to peer rejection, further exacerbating a child's social anxiety.

- Bullying and Teasing: Anxious children may become targets for bullying or teasing, which can worsen their anxiety and self-esteem.

2.1.3 Long-term Consequences

The effects of childhood anxiety can extend beyond the formative years, impacting a child's long-term well-being:

- Mental Health: Untreated childhood anxiety can increase the risk of developing other mental health disorders in adolescence and adulthood, such as depression, substance abuse, and more severe anxiety disorders.

- Self-esteem: Chronic anxiety can erode a child's self-esteem, making it challenging to develop a positive self-image and a strong sense of self-worth.

- Educational and Career Opportunities: The academic setbacks resulting from childhood anxiety can affect a child's future educational and career opportunities.

Recognizing the impact of childhood anxiety is the first step in understanding the urgency of intervention. By addressing anxiety in its early stages, we can help children build the emotional resilience and coping skills they need to overcome its challenges. In the chapters ahead, we'll explore strategies for providing effective support and guidance to children, empowering them to manage their anxiety and unlock their full potential.

2.2 Seeking Professional Help

Childhood anxiety is a significant concern that can have a profound impact on a child's well-being, development, and future success. While the support and understanding of parents, caregivers, and educators are crucial, it's essential to recognize that professional help can be a vital component of managing childhood anxiety effectively. In this section, we delve into the importance of seeking professional assistance when dealing with childhood anxiety, and we explore the different avenues available for support.

2.2.1 Pediatricians and Child Psychologists

Pediatricians and child psychologists are valuable resources for assessing and addressing childhood anxiety. Here's how they can assist:

- Pediatricians: Regular visits to a pediatrician are an opportunity for early detection of anxiety symptoms. Pediatricians can perform physical examinations, discuss developmental milestones, and provide guidance on managing common childhood concerns. They may also refer children to mental health specialists if necessary.

- Child Psychologists: Child psychologists are trained to assess and treat emotional and behavioral issues in children. They can conduct psychological assessments, diagnose anxiety disorders, and provide evidence-based therapies tailored to a child's specific needs. Cognitive-behavioral therapy (CBT) and play therapy are often used to help children manage their anxiety.

2.2.2 Therapeutic Approaches

Several therapeutic approaches have proven effective in helping children manage anxiety:

- Cognitive-Behavioral Therapy (CBT): CBT is a widely recognized and evidence-based therapy for childhood anxiety. It helps children identify and challenge irrational thoughts and beliefs that contribute to their anxiety. Through CBT, children learn coping strategies and problem-solving skills.

- Play Therapy: Play therapy is particularly useful for younger children who may have difficulty expressing their emotions verbally. In this approach, children use play as a medium to explore and communicate their feelings.

- Exposure Therapy: Exposure therapy involves gradually exposing children to anxiety-provoking situations in a controlled and supportive environment. Over time, this helps them build confidence and reduce anxiety related to specific triggers.

- Medication: In severe cases of childhood anxiety, when other interventions have not been effective, medication may be considered. Medications are typically prescribed and closely monitored by a child psychiatrist or pediatrician.

Chapter 3: Building a Supportive Environment

Introduction

In the journey to help children manage anxiety effectively, the importance of creating a supportive environment cannot be overstated. A nurturing and understanding environment can be the cornerstone of a child's emotional well-being, providing the stability and encouragement needed to confront and conquer anxiety challenges. In this chapter, we explore the fundamental elements of building a supportive environment for children grappling with anxiety.

Childhood anxiety is not a battle that children should have to face alone. It's a journey that involves the active participation of parents, caregivers, educators, and peers. By creating a supportive environment, we lay the foundation for children to develop resilience, self-confidence, and the skills necessary to manage their anxiety effectively.

We will delve into essential aspects of building this supportive atmosphere, including open communication, setting realistic expectations, and fostering self-care practices. By implementing these strategies, we aim to empower children with the tools they need to navigate their anxiety challenges while fostering a sense of security, trust, and love.

As we embark on this chapter, remember that supporting a child with anxiety is not about erasing anxiety entirely. Instead, it's about equipping them with the skills and confidence to face their worries and fears, knowing they have a reliable support system to lean on. Together, we can create an environment where children can thrive emotionally, socially, and academically, regardless of the anxiety challenges they may encounter along the way.

3.1.1 Creating a Safe Space

In the journey to support children with anxiety, one of the foundational elements is the creation of a safe and secure environment. A safe space is more than just a physical location; it's a psychological and emotional haven where children can feel protected, heard, and valued. This safe space serves as a crucial anchor for children as they navigate the often turbulent waters of anxiety.

Here are key components of creating a safe space for children dealing with anxiety:

1. Non-judgmental Atmosphere: A safe space should be free of judgment and criticism. Children need to know that they can express their thoughts, feelings, and concerns without fear of being ridiculed or belittled. Encourage open dialogue and active listening, where children feel heard and understood.

2. Trust and Confidentiality: Establish trust as the foundation of your relationship with the child. Children should feel confident that what they share in this safe space will remain confidential unless there is a legitimate concern for their safety. Respecting their privacy fosters trust and encourages open communication.

3. Predictability and Routine: Consistency and predictability can provide a sense of security for anxious children. Establish routines and clear boundaries within the safe space to help children understand what to expect. Knowing that there are reliable structures in place can reduce anxiety related to unpredictability.

4. Comfort and Physical Safety: Ensure that the physical environment of the safe space is comfortable and free from hazards. This includes making sure the child feels physically safe and can access any tools or resources they may need to manage their anxiety.

5. Emotional Validation: Validating a child's emotions is crucial in creating a safe space. Acknowledge their feelings, even if you don't fully understand them. Let them know that it's okay to feel the way they do and that their emotions are valid.

6. Encouragement and Positive Reinforcement: In a safe space, provide encouragement and positive reinforcement for efforts made to manage anxiety. Celebrate small victories and progress, no matter how minor they may seem. Positive feedback can boost a child's self-esteem and motivation.

7. Flexibility and Adaptability: Understand that the needs of anxious children can change over time. Be adaptable and willing to modify the safe space and support strategies to meet their evolving needs.

Creating a safe space is not a one-time effort; it's an ongoing commitment to providing a nurturing and understanding environment. When children know they have a safe space to turn to, it can significantly enhance their ability to cope with anxiety, build resilience, and develop the skills necessary to navigate life's challenges. In the chapters that follow, we will continue to explore additional ways to support anxious children within this safe and caring environment.

3.1.2 Active Listening

Active listening is a powerful tool in creating a supportive environment for children dealing with anxiety. It's more than just hearing words; it involves fully engaging with the child's thoughts and feelings, showing empathy, and providing them with your undivided attention. Active listening communicates to the child that their concerns and emotions are valued, fostering trust and strengthening the bond between you.

Here are essential aspects of active listening:

1. Give Your Full Attention: When a child seeks to communicate with you, set aside distractions and give them your full attention. This means putting away your phone, turning off the TV, and making eye contact to show that you are fully present.

2. Non-Verbal Cues: Your body language communicates a lot. Maintain an open posture, nod in agreement, and use facial expressions that convey understanding and empathy. These non-verbal cues reassure the child that you are genuinely listening.

3. Maintain Silence: Sometimes, silence is an essential part of active listening. Allow the child to express themselves without interruption. Give them the time they need to gather their thoughts and convey their feelings.

4. Reflect and Clarify: After the child has shared their thoughts or concerns, reflect back what you heard to ensure you understand correctly. For example, you can say, "I hear you saying that you're feeling really anxious about the upcoming test. Is that right?" This not only clarifies their feelings but also validates their experiences.

5. Ask Open-Ended Questions: Encourage the child to elaborate on their feelings and experiences by asking open-ended questions. Instead of yes-or-no questions, use inquiries like, "Can you tell me more about what's been bothering you lately?" These questions invite deeper sharing.

6. Avoid Judgment and Problem-Solving: Active listening is about creating a safe space for the child to express themselves, not about immediately solving their problems or passing judgment. Refrain from offering solutions or criticisms during the initial sharing. Your primary role is to listen and understand.

7. Empathize: Show empathy by acknowledging the child's feelings and expressing understanding. You can say, "I can imagine that must be really tough for you," or "I'm here for you, and I want to understand how you're feeling."

8. Validate Emotions: Let the child know that their emotions are valid, even if you don't share the same feelings. Avoid dismissing or minimizing their concerns. Validating their emotions can help them feel understood and accepted.

Active listening creates an environment where children feel heard, valued, and supported. It's a vital foundation for effective communication and emotional connection. When children know they can turn to you as a trusted listener, they are more likely to share their anxieties and concerns openly, making it easier to provide the support and guidance they need to manage their anxiety effectively.

3.2 Setting Realistic Expectations

Setting realistic expectations is a crucial aspect of building a supportive environment for children dealing with anxiety. By establishing reasonable and achievable goals and standards, you can help reduce stress and pressure, foster a sense of accomplishment, and create an atmosphere where children feel empowered rather than overwhelmed.

Here are important considerations when setting realistic expectations for anxious children:

1. Acknowledge Individual Differences: Recognize that each child is unique, and their abilities, strengths, and challenges may vary. Avoid comparing them to siblings or peers. Instead, focus on their individual progress and growth.

2. Understand Developmental Stages: Be mindful of age-appropriate expectations. Understand the typical developmental milestones for a child's age and adjust your expectations accordingly. Younger children may require more guidance and support, while older children may have increased responsibilities.

3. Balance Challenges and Support: Encourage children to step out of their comfort zones and face anxiety-provoking situations gradually. However, ensure that the challenges you introduce are manageable and not too overwhelming. Provide the necessary support and guidance to help them succeed.

4. Break Tasks into Smaller Steps: Complex tasks or goals can be daunting for anxious children. Break them down into smaller, more manageable steps. This approach allows children to experience a sense of accomplishment as they make progress.

5. Emphasize Effort Over Outcome: Shift the focus from the end result to the effort and dedication a child puts into a task or goal. Encourage a growth mindset, where mistakes are seen as opportunities to learn and improve.

6. Encourage Open Communication: Create an environment where children feel comfortable discussing their concerns and limitations. Encourage them to express when they feel overwhelmed or need adjustments to their expectations.

7. Promote Self-Care: Teach children the importance of self-care and the need to balance responsibilities with relaxation and downtime. Help them identify activities that help reduce anxiety and promote well-being.

8. Flexibility and Adaptation: Be flexible in adjusting expectations as circumstances change. Children may face unexpected challenges or setbacks, and it's essential to adapt expectations accordingly.

9. Celebrate Achievements: Celebrate both small and significant achievements. Recognize and praise the child's efforts, progress, and resilience. Positive reinforcement can boost self-esteem and

motivation.

10. Model Realistic Expectations: Children often learn by example. Model healthy and realistic expectations for yourself and others, demonstrating that it's okay to acknowledge limitations and seek support.

Setting realistic expectations is not about lowering standards but about creating an environment where children can thrive, build confidence, and manage anxiety effectively. By aligning your expectations with a child's developmental stage and individual needs, you provide them with the support and encouragement they require to face challenges and achieve success on their unique journey.

3.2.1 Balancing Academics and Extracurriculars

Balancing academics and extracurricular activities is a common challenge for children, and it's particularly relevant when supporting anxious children. While both areas are essential for a child's growth and development, finding the right equilibrium is crucial to prevent overwhelming anxiety and burnout. In this section, we explore how to strike a balance between academics and extracurriculars while accommodating an anxious child's needs.

1. Prioritize Well-Being: Start by emphasizing the importance of well-being over achievement. Let your child know that their physical and emotional health come first. Encourage open discussions about how they feel in different situations and help them recognize signs of stress or anxiety.

2. Assess Extracurricular Involvement: Evaluate the number and nature of extracurricular activities your child is engaged in. Consider their interests and passions, but also be mindful of the time and energy each activity demands. Limit the number of commitments to ensure there is ample downtime.

3. Set Realistic Academic Expectations: Work with your child's teachers to establish realistic academic expectations. Understand the curriculum and the pace at which your child is comfortable learning. Ensure that academic challenges are appropriate and manageable.

4. Create a Balanced Schedule: Help your child create a balanced weekly schedule that includes time for academics, extracurricular activities, relaxation, and sleep. Ensure that the schedule accommodates their anxiety-related needs, such as time for relaxation and coping strategies.

5. Encourage Time Management: Teach your child effective time management skills. Help them break tasks into smaller, manageable parts, set priorities, and plan their study and activity time effectively. Time management can reduce last-minute stress and anxiety.

6. Monitor Stress Levels: Keep a watchful eye on your child's stress levels. If you notice signs of excessive stress or anxiety, such as changes in behavior or physical symptoms, address them promptly. Adjust their schedule or seek professional guidance as needed.

7. Foster a Growth Mindset: Encourage a growth mindset by emphasizing that mistakes and setbacks are opportunities for learning and growth. Help your child understand that perfection is not the goal, and it's okay to make mistakes.

8. Communicate with Teachers and Coaches: Maintain open communication with your child's teachers and extracurricular coaches or instructors. Inform them of your child's anxiety-related needs and

collaborate to ensure that expectations and demands are reasonable.

9. Promote Self-Care: Teach your child the importance of self-care. Encourage relaxation techniques, exercise, and hobbies that help them unwind and recharge. Self-care is an essential tool for managing anxiety and maintaining balance.

10. Be Flexible: Be willing to adjust the balance between academics and extracurriculars as your child's needs change. Flexibility in scheduling and priorities ensures that your child can adapt to new challenges without becoming overwhelmed.

Balancing academics and extracurriculars is an ongoing process that requires regular assessment and adjustment. By prioritizing your child's well-being, setting realistic expectations, and promoting effective time management, you can create a supportive environment where they can flourish academically and enjoy their extracurricular pursuits without succumbing to excessive anxiety or stress.

3.2.2 Encouraging Self-Care

Encouraging self-care is a vital component of creating a supportive environment for children dealing with anxiety. Teaching children how to prioritize and care for their physical and emotional well-being equips them with essential tools for managing anxiety effectively. Here are key principles for fostering self-care practices in anxious children:

1. Model Self-Care: Children learn by example. Demonstrate self-care practices in your own life, such as maintaining a healthy work-life balance, engaging in relaxation activities, and seeking support when needed. Your actions serve as a powerful model for them to follow.

2. Educate About Self-Care: Talk to your child about the importance of self-care and its positive impact on mental and emotional well-being. Help them understand that self-care is not selfish but necessary for their overall health.

3. Identify Personal Self-Care Strategies: Work with your child to identify self-care strategies that resonate with them. These can include activities like reading, drawing, playing music, journaling, engaging in physical exercise, or spending time in nature. Tailor self-care practices to your child's interests and preferences.

4. Schedule Regular Self-Care Time: Incorporate dedicated self-care time into your child's daily or weekly routine. This time should be protected and seen as a non-negotiable part of their schedule. Encourage them to use this time to engage in their chosen self-care activities.

5. Teach Stress Reduction Techniques: Teach your child simple stress reduction techniques, such as deep breathing exercises, progressive muscle relaxation, or mindfulness meditation. These techniques can help them manage anxiety in real-time.

6. Encourage Healthy Habits: Promote healthy lifestyle habits, including regular exercise, a balanced diet, and adequate sleep. These habits have a direct impact on a child's physical and emotional well-being.

7. Set Boundaries: Help your child establish boundaries when it comes to their commitments and

responsibilities. Teach them to say "no" when they feel overwhelmed or when additional commitments may compromise their self-care.

8. Support Seeking Help: Encourage your child to seek help and support when needed. Let them know that it's okay to talk to a trusted adult or mental health professional if they are struggling with anxiety.

9. Monitor Self-Care Habits: Keep an eye on your child's self-care habits and well-being. Check in with them regularly to ensure they are taking time for self-care and coping effectively with anxiety-related challenges.

10. Celebrate Self-Care Achievements: Celebrate your child's self-care achievements, no matter how small. Recognize their efforts to prioritize self-care and acknowledge the positive impact it has on their anxiety management.

Fostering self-care practices empowers children to take an active role in their own well-being and provides them with effective tools for managing anxiety. By integrating self-care into their daily lives and promoting its benefits, you help create a supportive environment where they can thrive emotionally and build resilience in the face of anxiety.

Chapter 4: Coping Strategies for Kids

Introduction

Helping children develop effective coping strategies is a cornerstone of supporting them in their journey to manage anxiety. Coping strategies are the tools and techniques that children can use to navigate life's challenges, reduce stress, and confront anxiety-related difficulties. In this chapter, we explore a range of coping strategies tailored specifically for children, offering practical guidance for parents, caregivers, educators, and children themselves.

Childhood can be a time of intense emotions and significant life changes, making the development of coping skills crucial. While it's natural for children to experience anxiety from time to time, it's equally important for them to learn how to cope with and overcome these feelings. By equipping them with effective coping strategies, we empower children to face adversity with resilience and confidence.

In the chapters that follow, we will delve into various coping strategies designed to help children manage their anxiety. These strategies encompass emotional regulation, problem-solving, relaxation techniques, and social support. By understanding and implementing these techniques, children can build a toolkit of skills that will serve them well throughout their lives.

As we explore these coping strategies, keep in mind that each child is unique, and what works for one may not work for another. It's essential to adapt these strategies to suit the individual needs and preferences of the child. Together, we will embark on a journey to empower children with the skills they need to conquer anxiety and thrive emotionally, socially, and academically.

4.1 Mindfulness and Relaxation Techniques

Mindfulness and relaxation techniques are powerful tools that can help children manage anxiety by promoting a sense of calm, reducing stress, and enhancing self-awareness. These techniques empower children to stay present in the moment, acknowledge their feelings without judgment, and develop a greater sense of control over their emotions. In this section, we explore mindfulness and relaxation strategies tailored specifically for children.

4.1.1 Deep Breathing Exercises

Deep breathing exercises are simple yet effective relaxation techniques that can help children manage anxiety and stress. These exercises promote relaxation by slowing down the heart rate, calming the nervous system, and increasing oxygen flow to the brain. Teaching children how to engage in deep breathing can empower them with a valuable tool to use whenever they need to regain composure and reduce anxiety.

Here are steps to introduce deep breathing exercises to children:

1. Find a Comfortable Position: Encourage the child to sit or lie down in a comfortable and relaxed position. They can sit cross-legged on the floor or in a chair with their feet flat on the ground and hands resting on their lap.

2. Explain the Exercise: Explain to the child that deep breathing involves taking slow and deep breaths to relax their body and mind. You can use simple language like, "We're going to practice taking big, calm breaths to help us feel better."

3. Focus on the Breath: Instruct the child to place one hand on their chest and the other on their abdomen. Ask them to pay attention to their breath and notice how their chest and abdomen rise and fall with each breath.

4. Take a Deep Breath In: Have the child take a slow, deep breath in through their nose, counting to three as they inhale. Encourage them to feel their abdomen rise as they fill their lungs with air.

5. Exhale Slowly: Instruct the child to exhale slowly and gently through their mouth, counting to three as they breathe out. They should feel their abdomen fall as they release the breath.

6. Repeat Several Times: Have the child repeat this deep breathing cycle several times. You can count together as a guide. For example, inhale for three counts, exhale for three counts, and repeat this process for several rounds.

7. Encourage Visualization: To make deep breathing more engaging, you can encourage the child to imagine they are filling their body with calm and positive energy as they inhale and releasing stress or worries as they exhale.

8. Practice Regularly: Encourage the child to practice deep breathing exercises regularly, especially when they feel anxious or stressed. The more they practice, the more effective this technique becomes.

9. Use Visual Aids: Younger children may benefit from using visual aids like a breathing buddy or a soft toy placed on their abdomen to rise and fall with their breath. This can make the exercise more interactive and fun.

Deep breathing exercises are versatile and can be used anywhere, making them a valuable tool for children to manage anxiety in various situations. By incorporating deep breathing into their daily routine, children can develop the skills to calm their minds, reduce anxiety, and regain control over their emotions.

4.1.2 Guided Imagery

Guided imagery is a relaxation technique that encourages children to use their imagination to create calming mental images. This technique can help children manage anxiety by diverting their focus from worrisome thoughts and feelings to a more peaceful and positive mental space. Guided imagery is a valuable tool for promoting relaxation and emotional well-being in children. Here's how to introduce guided imagery to them:

1. Find a Quiet Space: Start by finding a quiet and comfortable space where the child can sit or lie down. Ensure that there are minimal distractions.

2. Set the Scene: Begin by describing a peaceful and calming scene to the child. For example, you can say, "Imagine you are on a beautiful, sunny beach. The sky is clear, and you can hear the gentle sound of waves."

3. Engage the Senses: Encourage the child to engage all their senses in their imagination. Ask them to visualize what they see, hear, smell, taste, and feel in this peaceful place. Encourage them to make the mental image as vivid as possible.

4. Use Positive Language: Throughout the guided imagery, use positive and soothing language. Describe the scene in a way that promotes relaxation and emotional well-being.

5. Encourage Deep Breathing: Combine guided imagery with deep breathing. Instruct the child to take slow, deep breaths as they immerse themselves in their mental image. For example, "As you inhale, feel the warm sun on your skin, and as you exhale, let go of any tension."

6. Visualize Stress Reduction: Prompt the child to visualize the stress or anxiety they may be feeling as a physical object, like a balloon or a cloud. Encourage them to imagine this object gradually floating away, becoming smaller and smaller.

7. Allow Exploration: Give the child some time to explore their peaceful mental scene. Let them use their imagination to interact with their surroundings in a way that brings comfort and relaxation.

8. Return to Reality: When the child is ready, gently guide them back to the present moment. You can do this by counting slowly from one to five, letting them know that when you reach five, they will open their eyes and return to their surroundings.

9. Reflect and Discuss: After the guided imagery, take a moment to discuss the experience with the child. Ask them how they felt and what they enjoyed about the mental journey.

10. Practice Regularly: Encourage the child to practice guided imagery regularly, especially when they are feeling anxious or stressed. With consistent practice, they can use this technique to find moments of peace and relaxation whenever needed.

Guided imagery is a creative and effective way for children to manage anxiety and promote emotional well-being. It allows them to tap into the power of their imagination to create a mental sanctuary where they can find comfort and calmness, even in challenging moments.

4.2 Cognitive Behavioral Techniques

Cognitive Behavioral Techniques (CBT) are evidence-based strategies that can help children manage anxiety by identifying and challenging negative thought patterns and behaviors. CBT is a structured and goal-oriented approach that empowers children to recognize, understand, and modify their thoughts and reactions to anxiety-inducing situations. Here, we explore CBT techniques specifically tailored for children:

4.2.1 Identifying Negative Thoughts

Identifying negative thoughts is a fundamental step in Cognitive Behavioral Techniques (CBT) for managing anxiety in children. It involves helping children become aware of the thoughts that contribute to their anxiety and recognizing the patterns of thinking that may be irrational or unhelpful. By identifying these negative thoughts, children can gain better control over their anxiety and work towards more rational and constructive thinking.

How to Implement Identifying Negative Thoughts:

1. Encourage Self-Awareness: Teach children to pay attention to their thoughts when they are feeling anxious or stressed. Explain that thoughts have a significant impact on emotions and behaviors.

2. Create a Thought Journal: Have children keep a "thought journal" or diary where they can record their anxious thoughts. Instruct them to note the date, time, and situation that triggered the thought.

3. Identify Specific Thoughts: Ask children to describe the thoughts that crossed their minds during anxious moments. Encourage them to be as specific as possible in identifying these thoughts.

4. Recognize Patterns: Help children recognize recurring themes or patterns in their negative thoughts. Are there certain situations or triggers that consistently lead to anxiety?

5. Challenge Negative Thoughts: Once negative thoughts are identified, guide children in challenging these thoughts. Encourage them to ask questions like, "Is this thought based on facts?" or "What evidence supports or refutes this thought?"

6. Label Distortions: Teach children about common cognitive distortions, such as all-or-nothing thinking, catastrophizing, or mind-reading. Help them recognize when these distortions appear in their thoughts.

7. Replace with Rational Thoughts: Work with children to replace negative or irrational thoughts with more balanced and rational alternatives. Encourage them to reframe their thinking to be more constructive and realistic.

8. Practice Regularly: Emphasize the importance of regular practice in identifying and challenging negative thoughts. The more children practice, the more proficient they become in recognizing and managing their anxious thinking.

Identifying negative thoughts is a crucial skill that equips children with the ability to take control of their thought patterns and reduce anxiety. By teaching them to recognize, challenge, and replace negative thoughts, you empower them to develop healthier thinking habits and build resilience in the face of anxiety.

4.2.2 Positive Self-Talk

Positive self-talk is a powerful Cognitive Behavioral Technique (CBT) that helps children manage anxiety by changing the way they speak to themselves internally. It involves replacing negative and self-critical thoughts with positive, supportive, and constructive messages. Positive self-talk can boost self-esteem, increase confidence, and reduce anxiety by promoting a more optimistic and self-compassionate mindset.

How to Implement Positive Self-Talk:

1. Raise Awareness: Teach children to become aware of their inner dialogue—the thoughts and messages they tell themselves in various situations, especially when they feel anxious or stressed.

2. Identify Negative Self-Talk: Encourage children to identify and label negative or unhelpful self-talk. These may include self-criticism, self-doubt, or overly negative assessments of situations.

3. Challenge Negative Thoughts: Help children challenge their negative self-talk by asking questions like, "Is this thought based on facts?" or "What evidence supports or refutes this thought?"

4. Replace with Positive Messages: Guide children in replacing negative thoughts with positive, constructive messages. Encourage them to use affirmations or statements that promote self-confidence and optimism.

5. Offer Supportive Phrases: Provide children with supportive phrases they can use during moments of anxiety. Examples include, "I can handle this," "I am capable," or "I have faced challenges before, and I can overcome this one."

6. Practice Self-Compassion: Teach children to be kind and compassionate toward themselves. Help them understand that making mistakes or facing difficulties is a natural part of life, and it doesn't diminish their worth.

7. Visualize Success: Encourage children to visualize themselves successfully managing anxiety-inducing situations. This mental rehearsal can boost their confidence and resilience.

8. Reinforce Positivity: Praise and reinforce positive self-talk when you hear your child using it. Celebrate their efforts to change their internal dialogue.

9. Create Positive Affirmations: Work with children to create their own positive affirmations that are tailored to their specific anxiety triggers. These affirmations should be personal, meaningful, and easy to remember.

10. Use Positive Self-Talk Daily: Emphasize the importance of daily practice. Positive self-talk is most effective when it becomes a regular habit. Encourage children to use it not only during anxious moments but also as a part of their daily routine.

Positive self-talk is a valuable skill that empowers children to reframe their thoughts and emotions in a more positive and constructive light. By incorporating positive messages into their self-talk, children can boost their self-esteem, reduce anxiety, and develop greater resilience in facing life's challenges.

Chapter 5: Healthy Lifestyle Habits

Introduction

In our journey to help children manage anxiety, it's essential to recognize the profound impact that lifestyle habits have on their overall well-being. Chapter 5 focuses on cultivating healthy lifestyle habits that promote physical, emotional, and mental health in children. These habits serve as a strong foundation for anxiety management and provide children with the resilience and vitality needed to navigate life's ups and downs.

Childhood is a critical period for developing healthy habits that can last a lifetime. By instilling these habits early on, we empower children to not only manage anxiety effectively but also thrive in all aspects of their lives. From nutrition and exercise to sleep and screen time, this chapter delves into the key areas that contribute to a child's overall health and well-being.

As parents, caregivers, educators, and role models, it is our responsibility to guide and support children in adopting and maintaining these healthy lifestyle habits. By doing so, we contribute to their emotional strength, self-confidence, and the tools they need to face anxiety with resilience.

In the pages that follow, we will explore various aspects of a healthy lifestyle and provide practical guidance on how to incorporate these habits into a child's daily routine. Together, we will embark on a journey to empower children with the knowledge and skills needed to lead a balanced, healthy, and anxiety-resistant life.

5.1 The Connection Between Diet and Anxiety

Diet plays a significant role in a child's physical health, but it also has a profound impact on their mental and emotional well-being. In this section, we delve into the intricate connection between diet and anxiety in children, highlighting how the foods they consume can influence their anxiety levels and overall emotional health.

5.1.1 Nutrient-Rich Foods

Nutrient-rich foods are the cornerstone of a healthy diet that can have a positive impact on a child's physical and mental well-being, including their ability to manage anxiety effectively. These foods are packed with essential vitamins, minerals, antioxidants, and other nutrients that support brain health and emotional resilience. Here are some key nutrient-rich foods that should be part of a child's diet:

1. Fruits and Vegetables: These are rich in vitamins, minerals, and antioxidants that support overall health. Encourage your child to eat a variety of colorful fruits and vegetables to ensure they get a wide range of nutrients.

2. Fatty Fish: Fatty fish like salmon, mackerel, and sardines are excellent sources of omega-3 fatty acids, which have been associated with reduced anxiety and improved mood.

3. Whole Grains: Whole grains like brown rice, whole wheat bread, and oatmeal provide complex

carbohydrates that help stabilize blood sugar levels and promote steady energy throughout the day.

4. Nuts and Seeds: Almonds, walnuts, flaxseeds, and chia seeds are rich in healthy fats, fiber, and nutrients that support brain health and emotional well-being.

5. Lean Proteins: Lean sources of protein like chicken, turkey, tofu, and legumes (beans and lentils) provide essential amino acids for neurotransmitter production, which can influence mood and anxiety.

6. Dairy or Dairy Alternatives: Dairy products (or fortified dairy alternatives) like yogurt, milk, and cheese are sources of calcium and vitamin D, which are important for bone health and may play a role in mood regulation.

7. Eggs: Eggs are a nutrient powerhouse, providing high-quality protein, essential vitamins, and minerals, including choline, which is important for brain function.

8. Leafy Greens: Leafy greens such as spinach, kale, and Swiss chard are rich in folate and other nutrients that support brain health and emotional well-being.

9. Berries: Berries like blueberries, strawberries, and raspberries are packed with antioxidants that may have mood-boosting properties.

10. Avocado: Avocado is a source of healthy fats and contains folate, which may play a role in reducing symptoms of depression and anxiety.

11. Fermented Foods: Fermented foods like yogurt, kefir, and kimchi contain probiotics that support gut health, which is increasingly linked to mental health.

12. Water: Staying properly hydrated is essential for overall health, including cognitive function and mood regulation. Encourage your child to drink water throughout the day.

Incorporating a variety of nutrient-rich foods into your child's diet can provide them with the essential building blocks for physical and emotional well-being. These foods support brain function, help stabilize mood, and contribute to overall resilience in the face of anxiety. Encourage your child to embrace a diverse and colorful diet to reap the benefits of these nutrient-rich options.

5.1.2 Limiting Sugar and Caffeine

While nutrient-rich foods are essential for supporting a child's mental and emotional well-being, it's equally important to be mindful of certain dietary components that can exacerbate anxiety. Two of these components are sugar and caffeine. Understanding the impact of these substances and implementing limits can contribute to better anxiety management in children.

5.1.2.1 The Effects of Sugar on Anxiety

Excessive sugar consumption, especially in the form of added sugars and sugary beverages, can have several negative effects on a child's mental health, including:

1. Blood Sugar Fluctuations: Sugary foods and drinks can cause rapid spikes and crashes in blood sugar levels, leading to mood swings and irritability, which can exacerbate anxiety.

2. Inflammation: A diet high in sugar can promote inflammation in the body, including the brain. Chronic inflammation has been linked to an increased risk of anxiety and other mood disorders.

3. Energy Levels: While sugar may provide a temporary energy boost, it's often followed by a "sugar crash" that can leave children feeling fatigued, irritable, and anxious.

4. Emotional Eating: Consuming sugary snacks in response to stress or anxiety can create a cycle of emotional eating, where sugar becomes a coping mechanism rather than a source of nourishment.

5.1.2.2 The Impact of Caffeine on Anxiety

Caffeine, commonly found in coffee, tea, energy drinks, and some sodas, is a stimulant that can affect anxiety levels in children. Here's how caffeine can contribute to anxiety:

1. Increased Heart Rate: Caffeine can lead to an elevated heart rate and feelings of jitteriness, which may mimic the physical sensations of anxiety.

2. Sleep Disruption: Consuming caffeine, especially in the afternoon or evening, can interfere with sleep quality. Sleep disturbances can exacerbate anxiety symptoms.

3. Heightened Stress Response: Caffeine can amplify the body's stress response, making children more reactive to stressors and potentially increasing feelings of anxiety.

4. Dependence: Regular caffeine consumption can lead to tolerance, meaning children may need more caffeine to achieve the same effects. This can result in withdrawal symptoms when caffeine is not consumed, including irritability and anxiety.

5.1.2.3 Practical Tips for Limiting Sugar and Caffeine

To promote better anxiety management in children, consider the following practical tips for limiting sugar and caffeine in their diets:

1. Read Labels: Pay attention to food and beverage labels to identify added sugars and opt for products with lower sugar content.

2. Offer Alternatives: Replace sugary snacks and drinks with healthier alternatives like fruit, whole-grain snacks, and water.

3. Set Limits: Establish guidelines for sugar and caffeine consumption in your household, and communicate these limits to your child.

4. Educate and Involve: Teach your child about the effects of sugar and caffeine on their bodies and emotions. Involve them in making healthier food and beverage choices.

5. Monitor Caffeine Intake: Be aware of your child's caffeine intake, especially from sources like

energy drinks and sodas. Limit their access to high-caffeine beverages.

6. Encourage Water: Encourage your child to drink water as their primary beverage to stay hydrated without the added effects of sugar and caffeine.

By limiting sugar and caffeine intake in your child's diet, you can create a foundation for better anxiety management. These dietary changes can help stabilize mood, reduce irritability, and promote emotional well-being, ultimately contributing to a healthier and more resilient child.

5.2 The Role of Exercise in Anxiety Management

Physical activity is a powerful tool for managing anxiety in children, offering numerous physical, emotional, and cognitive benefits. In this section, we explore the essential role of exercise in anxiety management and how it can positively impact a child's mental and emotional well-being.

5.2.1 Fun Physical Activities for Kids

Engaging in physical activities is not only important for a child's physical health but also for their emotional well-being. Encouraging fun and enjoyable physical activities can make exercise a positive and sustainable part of a child's routine. Here are some exciting physical activities that kids can enjoy while reaping the benefits of anxiety management:

1. Outdoor Play: Unstructured outdoor play allows kids to run, jump, climb, and explore. Activities like tag, hide and seek, and playing on playground equipment are excellent choices.

2. Biking: Riding a bicycle is a fantastic way to get exercise while having fun. Explore local bike paths or take family rides around the neighborhood.

3. Dancing: Crank up the music and have a dance party at home. Dancing is not only great exercise but also a mood booster.

4. Swimming: Swimming is not only a full-body workout but also a refreshing and enjoyable activity, especially during the summer months.

5. Sports: Enroll your child in a sports league or introduce them to sports like soccer, basketball, or tennis. Team sports provide exercise and social interaction.

6. Obstacle Courses: Set up an obstacle course in your backyard or at a local park using cones, ropes, and other materials. Challenge your child to complete the course while having fun.

7. Yoga: Children's yoga classes or online videos designed for kids can introduce them to the benefits of yoga, including relaxation and flexibility.

8. Hiking: Exploring nature on hikes is not only physically rewarding but also mentally rejuvenating. Look for family-friendly hiking trails in your area.

9. Rollerblading or Skateboarding: If your child enjoys these activities, they provide an excellent workout for balance and coordination.

10. Active Games: Games like Simon says, freeze tag, or hopscotch can get kids moving and having a blast.

11. Gardening: Gardening is a hands-on outdoor activity that involves digging, planting, and maintaining plants. It's a great way to connect with nature while staying active.

12. Family Walks: Take regular family walks around your neighborhood or local park. It's an opportunity to bond while staying active together.

13. Indoor Play Centers: On days when outdoor play isn't an option, consider indoor play centers that offer activities like trampolining or climbing walls.

14. Pretend Play: Encourage imaginative play that involves physical activity, such as pretending to be animals, superheroes, or explorers on a quest.

15. DIY Obstacle Course: Create a DIY obstacle course in your backyard or living room using cushions, pillows, and household items.

The key to making physical activity enjoyable for kids is to let them choose activities that interest them and to make it a family affair whenever possible. By promoting fun and active play, you not only support their physical health but also provide them with valuable tools for managing anxiety and stress in a positive way.

5.2.2 The Power of Play

Play is a child's natural and instinctive way of exploring the world, expressing themselves, and learning essential life skills. It's a powerful tool for managing anxiety, promoting emotional well-being, and developing resilience. In this section, we delve into the significance of play in helping children cope with anxiety and stress.

5.2.2.1 Play as a Stress Reliever

Play provides children with a healthy outlet to release pent-up energy and emotional tension. When they engage in play, whether it's imaginative play, active play, or creative play, they can experience the following stress-relieving benefits:

1. Emotional Expression: Play allows children to express their feelings, fears, and anxieties in a safe and non-judgmental way. They can act out scenarios and process their emotions through play.

2. Relaxation: Play promotes relaxation and reduces the physiological responses to stress, such as muscle tension and increased heart rate.

3. Distraction: Engaging in play can divert a child's attention away from worrisome thoughts and redirect their focus to the present moment.

4. Social Connection: Play often involves interaction with peers or family members, fostering social connections that provide emotional support and reduce feelings of isolation.

5.2.2.2 Types of Play for Anxiety Management

Different types of play can be particularly effective in helping children manage anxiety:

1. Imaginative Play: Role-playing, storytelling, and pretend play allow children to explore their emotions and fears in a safe and controlled environment. They can act out scenarios and develop problem-solving skills.

2. Active Play: Physical activities like running, jumping, climbing, and sports not only provide exercise but also release endorphins, which are natural mood lifters.

3. Creative Play: Engaging in artistic and creative activities, such as drawing, painting, crafting, or building, can be a calming and meditative way to express emotions.

4. Outdoor Play: Nature and outdoor environments offer a sense of calm and connection to the natural world. Outdoor play can reduce stress and promote well-being.

5. Social Play: Interacting with peers through play helps children build social skills, develop empathy, and create a support network.

5.2.2.3 Nurturing Playful Environments

To harness the power of play for anxiety management, create an environment that encourages and supports play:

1. Provide Play Materials: Offer a variety of toys, games, and materials that spark creativity and imagination.

2. Limit Screen Time: Reduce screen time to ensure that children have ample opportunities for unstructured play.

3. Participate Together: Join in on playtime with your child. Be an active participant and engage in imaginative scenarios or outdoor activities.

4. Encourage Free Play: Allow unstructured and free play where children can choose their activities and follow their interests.

5. Respect Play Choices: Honor your child's choices and preferences in play, even if they differ from your own.

6. Create a Playful Routine: Integrate playtime into your daily routine, ensuring that it becomes a regular and enjoyable part of your child's day.

7. Celebrate Creativity: Praise and celebrate your child's creative endeavors and imaginative play. Provide positive reinforcement for their efforts.

Play is a valuable and natural way for children to manage anxiety, reduce stress, and develop emotional resilience. By fostering a playful environment and actively participating in their play experiences, you empower your child with a powerful tool for coping with the challenges of anxiety.

Chapter 6: Managing Anxiety at School

Introduction

School is a crucial part of a child's life, where they learn, grow, and form lasting friendships. It's also a place where anxiety can manifest in various ways, affecting a child's academic performance, social interactions, and overall well-being. Chapter 6 delves into the essential strategies for managing anxiety at school, offering guidance to parents, caregivers, and educators on how to support children in this critical environment.

Anxiety at school can take on many forms, from test anxiety and social anxiety to separation anxiety and generalized anxiety. These challenges can impact a child's ability to learn, participate, and thrive in the classroom. Recognizing and addressing anxiety at school is essential to ensure that every child has the opportunity to reach their full potential.

In this chapter, we explore practical techniques for identifying anxiety in school-age children, providing appropriate support, and fostering a school environment that promotes emotional well-being. Whether your child is experiencing school-related anxiety or you are an educator seeking to create a more supportive classroom, the insights and strategies provided here aim to empower children to navigate the school experience with confidence and resilience.

By collaborating with teachers, school staff, and mental health professionals, we can create a nurturing and inclusive school environment where children can manage anxiety effectively, succeed academically, and enjoy their educational journey. Together, we can ensure that school is a place where every child can thrive.

6.1 Talking to Teachers and School Counselors

Open and effective communication with teachers and school counselors is a crucial step in managing anxiety at school. When parents and school professionals work together, they can provide the necessary support to help children cope with anxiety effectively. In this section, we'll explore the importance of initiating a conversation with teachers and school counselors and how to do it effectively.

6.1.1 Individualized Education Plans (IEPs)

An Individualized Education Plan, commonly referred to as an IEP, is a legally binding document designed to support students with disabilities, including those who experience anxiety or related challenges, in the educational setting. IEPs are customized plans tailored to a child's specific needs, ensuring that they receive the appropriate educational accommodations, services, and supports to succeed academically. Here's a closer look at the significance of IEPs for managing anxiety in school.

6.1.1.1 Identifying the Need for an IEP

An IEP is typically considered when a student's anxiety or related difficulties significantly impact their ability to access and make progress in the general education curriculum. Common signs that may lead to the consideration of an IEP for anxiety-related issues include:

- Frequent school avoidance or refusal due to anxiety.
- A pattern of academic decline resulting from anxiety.

- Consistent difficulty participating in classroom activities due to anxiety.
- The presence of a diagnosed anxiety disorder or other qualifying disability.

6.1.1.2 The IEP Development Process

Developing an IEP involves several key steps:

1. Referral and Assessment: The process begins with a referral, often initiated by parents, teachers, or school counselors, expressing concerns about a student's educational challenges due to anxiety. The school conducts a comprehensive assessment to determine the nature and extent of the student's needs.

2. IEP Team Meeting: A team, including parents or guardians, teachers, school counselors, special education professionals, and sometimes the student, convenes to discuss the assessment findings, identify goals, and determine appropriate accommodations and services.

3. Goal Setting: Specific, measurable, and achievable goals are established to address the student's needs related to anxiety. These goals guide the development of the IEP.

4. Accommodations and Services: The IEP outlines the accommodations and services the student will receive to support their anxiety management and academic success. These may include extra time on tests, access to a quiet space, counseling services, or the presence of a trusted adult.

5. Monitoring and Review: The IEP is a dynamic document that is periodically reviewed and adjusted as needed to ensure it remains relevant and effective for the student.

6.1.1.3 The Role of the IEP in Managing Anxiety

IEPs play a critical role in managing anxiety in school by providing:

- Accommodations: IEPs specify accommodations that can help alleviate anxiety-related barriers to learning. For instance, allowing a student more time to complete assignments or tests can reduce the pressure they feel.

- Support Services: IEPs may include access to support services such as counseling, which can provide strategies for managing anxiety and enhancing emotional well-being.

- Individualized Goals: Goals within the IEP are tailored to address specific anxiety-related challenges, ensuring that the student's progress is closely monitored and supported.

- Legal Protection: IEPs offer legal protections that ensure students receive the services and accommodations they need to access an appropriate education.

- Collaboration: The IEP process fosters collaboration among parents, teachers, counselors, and other professionals, creating a team focused on the student's success.

When anxiety significantly impacts a student's educational experience, an IEP can be a valuable tool for addressing their needs, reducing stress, and creating a supportive school environment where they can thrive academically and emotionally.

6.1.2 Reducing Academic Pressure

Academic pressure can exacerbate anxiety in students, making it essential to create a school environment that minimizes stress and supports emotional well-being. Reducing academic pressure can significantly benefit children with anxiety-related challenges. Here, we explore strategies for achieving this important goal.

6.1.2.1 Recognizing the Impact of Academic Pressure

Academic pressure often stems from high expectations, a focus on grades, and the fear of failure. It can manifest in various ways, including test anxiety, perfectionism, and a constant need for academic achievement. This pressure can take a toll on a child's mental health, leading to increased anxiety and decreased motivation to learn.

6.1.2.2 Strategies to Reduce Academic Pressure

To help manage anxiety at school, consider these strategies for reducing academic pressure:

1. Encourage a Growth Mindset: Promote the idea that intelligence and abilities can be developed through effort and learning. Emphasize the value of mistakes as opportunities for growth.

2. Set Realistic Expectations: Ensure that expectations for academic performance are realistic and tailored to the child's abilities and needs. Avoid setting unattainable goals.

3. Foster a Supportive Learning Environment: Create a classroom atmosphere where students feel comfortable asking questions, seeking help, and making mistakes without fear of judgment.

4. Emphasize Learning over Grades: Shift the focus from achieving high grades to valuing the process of learning. Encourage a love of learning for its own sake.

5. Offer Flexibility: Allow students flexibility in how they demonstrate their understanding, such as through alternative assessments or project-based learning.

6. Reduce Homework Overload: Consider age-appropriate homework loads and provide opportunities for students to practice skills without overwhelming them.

7. Teach Time Management: Help students develop effective time management skills to reduce last-minute cramming and stress.

8. Celebrate Effort and Progress: Recognize and celebrate students' hard work and progress rather than just the final outcome. Encourage a growth mindset.

9. Provide Test-Taking Support: Offer test-taking accommodations such as extended time, quiet spaces, or frequent breaks for students with test anxiety.

10. Promote Self-Care: Teach students about the importance of self-care, including getting enough sleep, maintaining a balanced diet, and engaging in physical activity.

11. Encourage Peer Support: Create opportunities for peer support and collaboration, which can reduce

feelings of isolation and competition.

12. Communicate Openly: Encourage students to communicate their concerns about academic pressure with teachers and counselors. Create a safe space for discussions about anxiety.

13. Offer Mindfulness Practices: Introduce mindfulness exercises and techniques that can help students manage stress and anxiety.

14. Involve Parents: Keep parents informed about classroom practices and provide resources for supporting their children at home.

By implementing these strategies, educators can help reduce academic pressure in the classroom, creating an environment where students can focus on learning, develop a positive attitude toward school, and effectively manage anxiety-related challenges.

6.2 Creating a Safe Space at School

One of the key elements in managing anxiety at school is the creation of a safe and supportive environment where students can feel secure, valued, and free to express themselves. In this section, we'll explore strategies for educators and schools to establish a safe space conducive to emotional well-being.

6.2.1 Peer Support

Peer support plays a vital role in creating a safe and inclusive environment at school, particularly for students dealing with anxiety or other emotional challenges. In this section, we'll explore the importance of peer support and strategies for promoting it within the school community.

6.2.1.1 The Significance of Peer Support

Peer support involves students helping and empathizing with their peers who may be experiencing anxiety, stress, or other emotional difficulties. Here's why peer support is essential:

1. Reduced Stigma: Peer support can help reduce the stigma surrounding mental health challenges, making it easier for students to seek help and share their experiences.

2. Shared Understanding: Peers often have a deeper understanding of what their classmates are going through, creating a strong sense of empathy and connection.

3. Increased Comfort: Students may feel more comfortable discussing their concerns with peers who share similar experiences, as opposed to adults.

4. Positive Influence: Peer support can positively influence behavior, encouraging students to seek help when needed and engage in pro-social behaviors.

6.2.1.2 Strategies for Promoting Peer Support

To promote peer support and create a nurturing environment at school, consider the following strategies:

1. Mentorship Programs: Implement mentorship programs where older students support younger ones, fostering a sense of belonging and guidance.

2. Peer Support Groups: Establish peer support groups or clubs where students can discuss their experiences and share coping strategies.

3. Training Workshops: Offer training workshops for students interested in becoming peer supporters, teaching active listening, empathy, and communication skills.

4. Buddy Systems: Implement buddy systems for new students, providing them with a peer who can help them adjust to the school environment.

5. Peer Education: Encourage students to educate their peers about mental health through presentations, workshops, or awareness campaigns.

6. Anonymous Reporting: Create anonymous reporting mechanisms for students to share concerns about bullying, harassment, or mental health issues.

7. Celebrate Diversity: Celebrate diversity and inclusivity to create a culture of acceptance and understanding among students.

8. Crisis Response Teams: Train selected students to be part of crisis response teams that can provide immediate support to peers in distress.

9. Peer Mediation: Train students in conflict resolution and mediation skills to help resolve conflicts among their peers.

10. Normalize Seeking Help: Encourage students to normalize seeking help from counselors, teachers, or trusted adults when they or their peers are struggling.

11. Student-Led Initiatives: Empower students to initiate and lead mental health awareness and support initiatives within the school.

12. Incorporate SEL: Integrate social-emotional learning (SEL) programs into the curriculum to teach students about empathy, self-awareness, and emotional regulation.

Peer support not only benefits students dealing with anxiety but also contributes to a more compassionate and understanding school community. By fostering an environment where peer support is encouraged and valued, schools can empower students to help each other navigate the challenges of anxiety and emotional well-being.

6.2.2 Stress-Free Study Tips

Effective study habits are essential for academic success, but they can also impact a student's stress levels. To create a safe and supportive learning environment, it's crucial to provide students with stress-free study tips. In this section, we'll explore strategies that educators and schools can promote to help students manage their anxiety while studying.

6.2.2.1 The Role of Stress-Free Study Habits

Stress-free study habits are essential because they:

1. Reduce Anxiety: By implementing stress-free strategies, students can reduce anxiety associated with studying, test preparation, and academic performance.

2. Enhance Learning: A relaxed and focused mind is more receptive to new information, leading to improved comprehension and retention of study material.

3. Promote Positive Attitudes: Stress-free study habits foster positive attitudes toward learning, encouraging students to view education as an enjoyable and fulfilling pursuit.

6.2.2.2 Strategies for Stress-Free Study

To promote stress-free study habits, educators and schools can emphasize the following strategies:

1. Time Management: Teach students effective time management techniques to prevent last-minute cramming and reduce study-related stress.

2. Break Tasks Into Smaller Steps: Encourage students to break down study tasks into smaller, manageable steps to prevent feeling overwhelmed.

3. Prioritize Self-Care: Remind students to prioritize self-care, including adequate sleep, a balanced diet, and regular physical activity, which can improve focus and reduce stress.

4. Create a Calm Study Environment: Help students establish a quiet and comfortable study space free from distractions.

5. Set Realistic Goals: Encourage students to set realistic and achievable study goals, rather than aiming for perfection.

6. Practice Mindfulness: Introduce mindfulness techniques, such as deep breathing or meditation, to help students stay calm and focused during study sessions.

7. Active Learning: Promote active learning strategies, such as summarizing, questioning, or teaching the material to others, which can enhance engagement and retention.

8. Utilize Resources: Make students aware of available study resources, including textbooks, online materials, and academic support services.

9. Encourage Breaks: Advise students to take short breaks during study sessions to prevent mental fatigue and improve concentration.

10. Practice Positive Self-Talk: Teach students to replace negative self-talk with positive affirmations, boosting their confidence and reducing anxiety.

11. Review Progress: Encourage students to regularly review their progress, celebrating their achievements and adjusting study strategies if necessary.

12. Seek Help When Needed: Promote a culture where students feel comfortable seeking help from teachers, tutors, or peers when they encounter challenging study material.

By incorporating stress-free study tips into the school culture and curriculum, educators can empower students to approach their studies with confidence, reduce anxiety, and foster a positive attitude toward learning. These strategies contribute to creating a safe and supportive academic environment that values students' well-being as much as their academic achievements.

Chapter 7: Nurturing Resilience and Self-esteem

Introduction

Resilience and self-esteem are two powerful tools that can help children not only cope with anxiety but also thrive in the face of life's challenges. In this chapter, we explore the essential role of resilience and self-esteem in a child's emotional well-being and provide guidance on how parents, caregivers, and educators can nurture these vital qualities.

Resilience is the ability to bounce back from adversity, overcome setbacks, and adapt to difficult situations. Self-esteem is the foundation of a child's self-worth and self-confidence. When children possess strong self-esteem and resilience, they are better equipped to navigate anxiety and stress, build positive relationships, and achieve their full potential.

In this chapter, we delve into practical strategies and exercises designed to help children develop resilience and bolster their self-esteem. By nurturing these qualities, we empower them to face anxiety head-on and emerge stronger, more confident, and better prepared for the challenges of life.

Resilience and self-esteem are not innate traits; they can be cultivated and strengthened through supportive environments, positive relationships, and intentional practices. As we explore these concepts in the chapters ahead, we invite you to embark on a journey of empowerment, guiding the children in your care toward a brighter, more resilient, and self-assured future.

7.1 Encouraging Problem-Solving Skills

Problem-solving skills are at the core of resilience and play a pivotal role in helping children effectively manage anxiety and life's challenges. In this section, we'll delve into the importance of nurturing problem-solving abilities and provide practical strategies for encouraging their development in children.

7.1.1 Facing Fears Gradually

Facing fears gradually, also known as systematic desensitization, is an evidence-based technique commonly used in cognitive-behavioral therapy (CBT) to help individuals, including children, manage and overcome anxiety. In this section, we explore the importance of facing fears gradually and how it can be applied effectively to support children dealing with anxiety.

7.1.1.1 Understanding Gradual Exposure

Gradual exposure is based on the principle that repeated, controlled exposure to anxiety-inducing situations or triggers can reduce fear and anxiety over time. It involves breaking down a feared situation or object into smaller, manageable steps or levels of exposure. Children are encouraged to confront these levels in a step-by-step fashion, gradually increasing the level of challenge as they become more comfortable.

7.1.1.2 The Benefits of Gradual Exposure

Facing fears gradually offers several benefits for children with anxiety:

1. Reduced Anxiety: It helps reduce anxiety by allowing children to approach feared situations at their own pace and in a controlled manner.

2. Increased Confidence: As children successfully confront their fears, their self-confidence and belief in their ability to cope with anxiety-inducing situations grow.

3. Improved Coping Skills: Gradual exposure teaches children effective coping skills, such as deep breathing and positive self-talk, which they can apply in various situations.

4. Long-Term Anxiety Reduction: It can lead to long-term anxiety reduction, as children learn to manage their fears independently.

7.1.1.3 Implementing Gradual Exposure

To implement gradual exposure effectively, consider the following steps:

1. Identify the Fear: Work with the child to identify their specific fear or anxiety trigger. This could be a situation, object, or activity.

2. Create a Hierarchy: Develop a fear hierarchy by listing levels of exposure from the least anxiety-provoking to the most anxiety-provoking. For example, if a child is afraid of dogs, the hierarchy might start with looking at pictures of dogs and progress to being near a small, calm dog.

3. Start at the Lowest Level: Begin with the lowest level of exposure, ensuring it is manageable and only slightly anxiety-inducing. For instance, if the child is afraid of public speaking, the initial exposure could be speaking in front of a trusted adult.

4. Practice Exposure: Encourage the child to practice exposure at the chosen level repeatedly until their anxiety decreases significantly.

5. Gradually Increase Difficulty: As the child becomes more comfortable, move to the next level of exposure in the hierarchy. Continue this process until they can confront the most anxiety-provoking situation or trigger.

6. Provide Support: Offer emotional support and reassurance throughout the process. Celebrate each success and acknowledge their courage.

7. Monitor Progress: Keep track of the child's progress and adjust the exposure plan as needed.

8. Seek Professional Help: In cases of severe anxiety or phobias, consider involving a mental health

professional who specializes in anxiety disorders to guide the gradual exposure process.

Gradual exposure is a valuable tool for helping children build resilience and manage anxiety. When implemented patiently and consistently, it can lead to significant improvements in their ability to confront and overcome their fears, ultimately enhancing their overall well-being.

7.1.2 Learning from Mistakes

Learning from mistakes is an essential aspect of helping children manage anxiety effectively. This section explores the importance of embracing mistakes as opportunities for growth and building resilience in anxious children.

7.1.2.1 Shifting the Perspective on Mistakes

For anxious children, mistakes can be a significant source of stress and anxiety. They often fear making errors in academic tasks, social interactions, or other aspects of their lives. Shifting the perspective on mistakes is crucial to help them manage anxiety more effectively.

7.1.2.2 The Benefits of Learning from Mistakes

Encouraging children to learn from mistakes offers several advantages:

1. Reduced Perfectionism: It helps reduce perfectionistic tendencies, where children feel they must avoid mistakes at all costs.

2. Increased Resilience: Learning from mistakes fosters resilience by teaching children that setbacks are a natural part of life and can be overcome.

3. Improved Problem-Solving Skills: Mistakes provide valuable learning opportunities, allowing children to develop problem-solving skills and adaptability.

4. Enhanced Self-Esteem: As children learn to handle mistakes and setbacks, their self-esteem and self-confidence grow.

7.1.2.3 Strategies for Embracing Mistakes

To help children embrace and learn from their mistakes, consider the following strategies:

1. Normalize Mistakes: Encourage a culture where making mistakes is seen as a normal and essential part of learning and growing.

2. Provide Constructive Feedback: Offer constructive feedback rather than criticism when children make mistakes. Focus on what they can learn from the experience.

3. Model Resilience: Demonstrate resilience by sharing your own experiences of making and learning from mistakes.

4. Encourage Problem-Solving: Guide children in analyzing their mistakes, helping them identify what went wrong and how they can improve next time.

5. Set Realistic Expectations: Encourage realistic expectations by emphasizing that nobody is perfect, and everyone makes mistakes.

6. Highlight Success Stories: Share stories of successful individuals who faced setbacks and learned from their mistakes on their path to success.

7. Celebrate Effort: Celebrate the effort children put into their tasks and activities, regardless of the outcome.

8. Encourage Reflection: Ask open-ended questions that encourage children to reflect on their experiences and what they have learned.

9. Support Self-Compassion: Teach children to be kind and compassionate toward themselves, even when they make mistakes.

10. Encourage Growth Mindset: Foster a growth mindset by emphasizing that abilities can be developed through effort and learning from mistakes.

Learning from mistakes can be a powerful tool in helping anxious children build resilience, reduce anxiety, and develop a healthier perspective on challenges. By embracing errors as opportunities for growth, children can approach life's ups and downs with greater confidence and a more positive outlook.

7.2 Building Self-Confidence

Building self-confidence is a fundamental aspect of helping children effectively manage anxiety. In this section, we explore the significance of self-confidence in anxiety management and strategies to nurture and strengthen it in children.

7.2.1 Celebrating Achievements

Celebrating achievements is a powerful way to boost children's self-confidence and foster a positive mindset. In this section, we'll explore the significance of celebrating achievements and how it contributes to anxiety management in children.

7.2.1.1 The Importance of Celebrating Achievements

Celebrating achievements serves as a catalyst for building self-confidence and managing anxiety because:

1. Positive Reinforcement: It provides positive reinforcement for a child's efforts, reinforcing the belief that their actions and hard work matter.

2. Increased Self-Esteem: Recognizing achievements boosts self-esteem, helping children view themselves in a more positive light.

3. Motivation: Celebrating accomplishments motivates children to set and pursue new goals, enhancing their sense of competence and self-efficacy.

4. Emotional Well-being: Regular celebrations contribute to a happier and more emotionally balanced child, reducing anxiety and stress.

7.2.1.2 Strategies for Celebrating Achievements

To effectively celebrate achievements and bolster self-confidence in children, consider the following strategies:

1. Acknowledge Effort: Recognize and celebrate the effort children put into their tasks and activities, emphasizing the value of hard work.

2. Set Milestones: Break larger goals into smaller milestones, making it easier for children to track their progress and celebrate smaller achievements along the way.

3. Be Specific: When praising an achievement, be specific about what was done well. Highlight the skills and qualities that led to success.

4. Create a Celebration Ritual: Establish a simple, personalized celebration ritual for each achievement, whether it's a high-five, a special treat, or a fun activity.

5. Encourage Self-Reflection: Prompt children to reflect on their accomplishments and what they have learned from the experience.

6. Involve Family and Friends: Share achievements with family and friends, encouraging positive reinforcement from loved ones.

7. Display Achievements: Create a visible display of achievements, such as a bulletin board or a wall of accomplishments, to remind children of their successes.

8. Journaling: Encourage children to keep a journal of their achievements, providing a tangible record of their progress.

9. Set Realistic Expectations: Ensure that the celebration aligns with the significance of the achievement. Reserve grand celebrations for major milestones and simple acknowledgments for smaller accomplishments.

10. Use Positive Language: Use positive and encouraging language when discussing achievements. Avoid comparisons with others.

11. Encourage Goal Setting: After celebrating one achievement, prompt children to set new goals to maintain motivation and a sense of purpose.

12. Foster a Growth Mindset: Emphasize that mistakes and setbacks are part of the learning process and that they can lead to future successes.

13. Be Consistent: Celebrate achievements consistently, whether they are academic, personal, or related to hobbies and interests.

Celebrating achievements not only boosts self-confidence but also reinforces a growth mindset, resilience, and a positive attitude toward challenges. It plays a pivotal role in helping children manage anxiety by building their belief in their abilities and fostering emotional well-being.

7.2.2 Embracing Uniqueness

Embracing uniqueness is a powerful strategy for building self-confidence in children and helping them effectively manage anxiety. In this section, we'll explore the importance of celebrating individuality and strategies to encourage children to embrace their uniqueness.

7.2.2.1 The Significance of Embracing Uniqueness

Embracing uniqueness is essential for anxiety management because:

1. Positive Self-Image: It promotes a positive self-image by helping children recognize and value their individual qualities, talents, and characteristics.

2. Self-Acceptance: Embracing uniqueness fosters self-acceptance, teaching children to be comfortable with who they are and reducing self-criticism.

3. Resilience: Children who embrace their uniqueness are often more resilient, as they have a strong sense of self and are less affected by external judgments and criticisms.

4. Reduces Peer Pressure: Embracing individuality can reduce the pressure to conform to peer expectations, helping children make choices based on their values and interests.

7.2.2.2 Strategies for Embracing Uniqueness

To encourage children to embrace their uniqueness and build self-confidence, consider the following strategies:

1. Encourage Self-Discovery: Support children in exploring their interests, passions, and talents to help them discover what makes them unique.

2. Celebrate Differences: Highlight the importance of diversity and celebrate differences among individuals, fostering an inclusive and accepting mindset.

3. Promote Self-Expression: Encourage self-expression through art, writing, music, or other creative outlets, allowing children to showcase their uniqueness.

4. Avoid Comparisons: Discourage comparisons with others and help children understand that everyone has their strengths and areas for growth.

5. Highlight Strengths: Emphasize and celebrate a child's strengths, talents, and achievements, no matter how big or small.

6. Encourage Authenticity: Teach children to be authentic and true to themselves, rather than trying to fit into prescribed molds or expectations.

7. Role Models: Share stories of individuals who have succeeded by embracing their uniqueness and staying true to themselves.

8. Address Bullying and Peer Pressure: Equip children with strategies to handle bullying and peer pressure, emphasizing the importance of standing up for their values.

9. Encourage Questions: Create an environment where children feel comfortable asking questions and seeking answers about their identity and uniqueness.

10. Build Self-Awareness: Help children develop self-awareness by encouraging them to reflect on their values, beliefs, and personal qualities.

11. Promote Inclusivity: Promote inclusivity and acceptance of all individuals, reinforcing the idea that diversity enriches our communities.

12. Be Supportive: Be a supportive and empathetic presence in a child's life, offering love and acceptance unconditionally.

Embracing uniqueness empowers children to build self-confidence, make choices that align with their values, and navigate life's challenges with authenticity and resilience. By encouraging children to celebrate their individuality, we equip them with the tools they need to effectively manage anxiety and develop a strong sense of self-worth.

Chapter 8: Coping with Specific Anxiety Challenges

Introduction

Anxiety is a complex and multifaceted emotion, and it manifests differently in each child. In this chapter, we delve into coping strategies tailored to address specific anxiety challenges that children may encounter in various aspects of their lives. Whether it's the fear of public speaking, social anxiety, or the stress of academic tests, we aim to provide practical guidance for parents, caregivers, and educators.

Understanding that anxiety is not a one-size-fits-all experience is crucial. Each child's anxiety challenges may be unique, influenced by their personality, life experiences, and individual triggers. It is our hope that the insights and strategies shared in this chapter will serve as a valuable resource for helping children navigate specific anxiety challenges effectively.

As we explore various anxiety scenarios and provide targeted coping techniques, we emphasize the importance of tailoring interventions to the child's specific needs. By addressing anxiety challenges head-on and equipping children with the right tools, we empower them to face their fears, build resilience, and live fulfilling lives despite anxiety's presence.

In the chapters that follow, we'll explore coping strategies for common anxiety scenarios, offering guidance and support to children and those who care for them. Together, we can help children conquer their anxiety challenges and embrace a brighter, more confident future.

8.1 Separation Anxiety

Separation anxiety is a common form of anxiety experienced by many children, typically during their early years. It manifests when children feel distressed or anxious when separated from their primary caregivers or familiar environments. This anxiety can be challenging for both children and parents, affecting daily routines, school transitions, and social interactions. In this section, we'll explore separation anxiety in depth, understanding its causes, signs, and strategies to help children cope with and overcome this common form of anxiety.

8.1.1 Transitioning Smoothly

Transitioning smoothly is a key component of managing separation anxiety in children. This subsection delves into the importance of well-managed transitions and provides strategies for parents, caregivers, and educators to help children cope with the anxiety associated with separations.

8.1.1.1 The Significance of Smooth Transitions

Well-managed transitions play a crucial role in alleviating separation anxiety because:

1. Predictability: Predictable transitions create a sense of security and reduce anxiety, as children know what to expect.

2. Trust: Consistently smooth transitions build trust between children and their caregivers or teachers, reducing anxiety about separations.

3. Emotional Preparation: Thoughtful transitions allow children to emotionally prepare for separations, making the process less daunting.

8.1.1.2 Strategies for Transitioning Smoothly

To facilitate smooth transitions and ease separation anxiety, consider implementing the following strategies:

1. Establish a Routine: Create a consistent daily routine with clear expectations and schedules for transitions.

2. Use Visual Cues: Visual schedules or timers can help children understand when separations will occur and how long they will last.

3. Offer Choices: Provide children with choices when appropriate, giving them a sense of control over their transitions.

4. Maintain Communication: Maintain open and reassuring communication with children about separations and reunions.

5. Gradual Separation: If possible, ease into separations gradually, starting with shorter periods and gradually increasing them.

6. Comfort Objects: Allow children to bring comfort objects, such as a favorite toy or blanket, to provide a sense of familiarity during separations.

7. Be Present: During transitions, be emotionally present with children, offering comfort, reassurance, and encouragement.

8. Develop a Goodbye Ritual: Create a special and consistent goodbye ritual that signals the start of a separation and assures the child of your return.

9. Engage in Positive Reunions: Celebrate reunions with enthusiasm and positivity, reinforcing the idea that separations are temporary.

10. Address Fears: If children express fears or concerns about separations, listen empathetically and provide honest, age-appropriate explanations.

11. Foster Independence: Encourage age-appropriate independence and self-reliance, helping children build confidence in their ability to handle separations.

12. Involve Teachers and Caregivers: Collaborate with teachers, caregivers, and other trusted adults to ensure consistency in managing transitions.

13. Practice Patience: Understand that separation anxiety is a normal part of childhood development, and it may take time for children to become more comfortable with separations.

Effective transitioning not only eases separation anxiety but also empowers children to develop the skills and resilience needed to navigate separations confidently. By implementing these strategies, caregivers and educators can create a supportive environment that helps children manage the challenges of separation more smoothly.

8.1.2 Building Trust

Building trust is a fundamental element in addressing separation anxiety in children. This subsection explores the significance of trust and offers strategies for parents, caregivers, and educators to establish and strengthen trust in children dealing with separation anxiety.

8.1.2.1 The Importance of Trust

Trust is a cornerstone in managing separation anxiety because:

1. Emotional Security: Trust provides children with a sense of emotional security, assuring them that their caregivers or teachers will return after a separation.

2. Predictability: Trust is closely tied to predictability, and children who trust that separations are temporary and safe are less likely to experience anxiety.

3. Resilience: Trust in the caregiver's or teacher's return builds resilience, helping children cope with separations and develop a positive attitude toward them.

8.1.2.2 Strategies for Building Trust

To foster trust and alleviate separation anxiety, consider implementing the following strategies:

1. Consistency: Maintain consistent routines, schedules, and expectations, which help children predict when separations will occur and when reunions will happen.

2. Honesty: Be honest and age-appropriate when discussing separations, explaining where you're going, when you'll return, and reinforcing that you'll always come back.

3. Follow Through: Always follow through on promises and commitments, reinforcing the trust that children have in your words and actions.

4. Be Responsive: Respond promptly and lovingly to children's needs and concerns, even when they express anxiety or sadness about separations.

5. Establish Reliability: Ensure that children can rely on you consistently for their basic needs and emotional support.

6. Predictable Goodbyes: Create a predictable and comforting goodbye routine that signals the start of a separation and reassures the child of your return.

7. Encourage Independence: Encourage age-appropriate independence and decision-making, allowing children to build trust in their own abilities.

8. Positive Reunions: Celebrate reunions with warmth and positivity, reinforcing the trust that separations are temporary.

9. Be Patient: Recognize that building trust takes time, especially for children with separation anxiety, and be patient in fostering this essential bond.

10. Build Trust with Caregivers and Teachers: Collaborate with caregivers and teachers to ensure consistency in building trust across different environments.

11. Acknowledge Feelings: Validate children's feelings of anxiety or sadness about separations, emphasizing that it's okay to feel this way and that you're there to support them.

12. Maintain Communication: Maintain open and reassuring communication with children, offering them opportunities to express their thoughts and feelings.

Building trust is an ongoing process that forms the foundation of a child's ability to cope with and eventually overcome separation anxiety. By consistently demonstrating trustworthiness and providing emotional support, caregivers and educators can help children feel secure and confident during separations.

8.2 Test and Performance Anxiety

Test and performance anxiety can affect children's academic performance and overall well-being. In this section, we'll explore the nuances of test and performance anxiety, its causes, and evidence-based strategies to help children manage these specific forms of anxiety. We'll address not only the immediate concerns related to exams and performances but also the long-term impact of anxiety on a child's self-esteem and academic success.

8.2.1 Effective Study Techniques

Effective study techniques are essential for managing test and performance anxiety in children. This subsection delves into the significance of adopting efficient study methods and provides strategies to help children prepare for tests and performances with confidence.

8.2.1.1 The Role of Effective Study Techniques

Utilizing effective study techniques is crucial for managing test and performance anxiety because:

1. Enhanced Preparedness: Effective study methods improve a child's preparedness for exams and performances, reducing anxiety related to feeling unprepared.

2. Confidence Building: When children are well-prepared, they feel more confident in their abilities, alleviating performance anxiety.

3. Improved Test-Taking Skills: Effective study techniques often include strategies for better test-taking skills, such as time management and stress reduction.

8.2.1.2 Strategies for Effective Study Techniques

To help children manage test and performance anxiety through effective study techniques, consider the following strategies:

1. Time Management: Teach children how to allocate their study time wisely, breaking down study sessions into manageable segments.

2. Active Learning: Encourage active learning techniques, such as summarizing, questioning, or teaching the material to others, which enhance engagement and retention.

3. Prioritization: Guide children in identifying key topics or concepts to prioritize during their study sessions, focusing on areas of greater importance.

4. Self-Quizzing: Incorporate self-quizzing or practice tests to help children assess their knowledge and build confidence.

5. Effective Note-Taking: Teach children effective note-taking skills during lectures or while reading textbooks to create useful study materials.

6. Mindful Study Breaks: Promote short, mindful study breaks during longer study sessions to prevent mental fatigue and maintain focus.

7. Goal Setting: Help children set specific study goals, making the study process more structured and rewarding.

8. Stress Reduction Techniques: Teach stress reduction techniques like deep breathing, mindfulness, and progressive muscle relaxation to manage anxiety during study sessions.

9. Consistency: Encourage consistent study habits by establishing a regular study schedule that includes

both daily review and long-term preparation.

10. Test Simulations: Familiarize children with test formats and conditions by simulating exam environments at home, including timed practice tests.

11. Seek Clarification: Encourage children to seek clarification from teachers or peers when they encounter challenging material.

12. Review Progress: Regularly review and assess their study progress, allowing them to adjust their strategies as needed.

13. Healthy Lifestyle: Promote a healthy lifestyle, including adequate sleep, balanced nutrition, and regular physical activity, which can improve focus and memory.

Effective study techniques not only help children perform better academically but also alleviate the anxiety associated with tests and performances. By teaching children these strategies and helping them integrate them into their study routines, caregivers and educators can empower them to approach exams and performances with confidence and reduced anxiety.

8.2.2 Relaxation Rituals

Relaxation rituals are valuable tools for helping children manage anxiety, especially when specific triggers or situations provoke heightened stress. In this section, we'll explore the concept of relaxation rituals and provide practical techniques that children can incorporate into their daily lives to alleviate anxiety.

8.2.2.1 The Role of Relaxation Rituals

Relaxation rituals serve several essential functions in anxiety management:

1. Stress Reduction: They help reduce the physiological and psychological symptoms of anxiety by promoting relaxation and calmness.

2. Anxiety Prevention: Regular practice of relaxation rituals can serve as a proactive approach to preventing anxiety before it becomes overwhelming.

3. Emotional Regulation: Relaxation techniques teach children to recognize and regulate their emotions, enhancing their ability to respond to anxiety-inducing situations with composure.

8.2.2.2 Strategies for Incorporating Relaxation Rituals

Encourage children to integrate relaxation rituals into their daily routines with these strategies:

1. Breathing Exercises: Teach children deep breathing exercises, like diaphragmatic breathing or the 4-7-8 technique, to calm their nervous system.

2. Mindfulness Meditation: Guide them through mindfulness meditation practices that focus on the present moment and alleviate anxiety-inducing thoughts.

3. Progressive Muscle Relaxation: Introduce progressive muscle relaxation, where they learn to systematically tense and release muscle groups to achieve physical relaxation.

4. Visualization: Encourage children to use guided imagery to imagine peaceful and safe places when feeling anxious.

5. Yoga and Stretching: Incorporate gentle yoga poses and stretching exercises to release physical tension.

6. Nature Connection: Spend time in nature, encouraging children to engage their senses in the calming effects of natural environments.

7. Artistic Expression: Engage in creative activities like drawing, coloring, or journaling to provide an outlet for emotions.

8. Music and Breathing: Use calming music in conjunction with deep breathing exercises to create a relaxing audio-visual experience.

9. Aromatherapy: Explore the use of calming scents, such as lavender or chamomile, through essential oils or diffusers.

10. Sensory Tools: Provide sensory tools like stress balls or fidget toys to help children redirect nervous energy.

11. Scheduled Relaxation Time: Set aside dedicated relaxation time in their daily schedule to ensure consistency.

12. Bedtime Rituals: Develop bedtime rituals that promote relaxation, such as reading a calming book or practicing deep breathing before sleep.

13. Positive Affirmations: Encourage the use of positive affirmations to challenge anxious thoughts and promote self-assurance.

14. Self-Monitoring: Teach children to recognize signs of anxiety and initiate relaxation rituals when needed.

By integrating relaxation rituals into a child's routine, we equip them with a set of practical tools to manage anxiety effectively. These rituals can be tailored to suit individual preferences, making them a versatile and empowering resource for children navigating specific anxiety challenges.

Chapter 9: Sibling and Family Dynamics

Introduction

Anxiety doesn't affect just the child who experiences it; it reverberates throughout the family, impacting sibling relationships, parental roles, and the overall family dynamic. In this chapter, we turn our attention to the complexities of sibling and family dynamics in the context of childhood anxiety. We aim to provide insights and strategies for parents and caregivers navigating these challenges while fostering a supportive and harmonious family environment.

Living with a sibling who experiences anxiety can be both rewarding and challenging. Siblings play a significant role in a child's life, and their interactions can influence emotional well-being. Understanding how to support both the anxious child and their siblings is crucial in maintaining family cohesion and nurturing each child's unique needs.

We recognize that parenting a child with anxiety often involves juggling the demands of school, therapy, and home life, which can strain family relationships. However, it's essential to remember that families have the potential to become a powerful source of support and resilience.

In the chapters ahead, we'll explore the intricacies of sibling relationships in the context of anxiety, offering guidance on promoting understanding, empathy, and collaboration among siblings. Additionally, we'll discuss effective communication strategies for parents and caregivers, helping them navigate the complexities of parenting multiple children with varying needs.

By addressing sibling and family dynamics, we aim to create a more empathetic and harmonious family unit where each member feels valued, understood, and equipped to support one another in managing anxiety challenges. Together, we can build a stronger, more resilient family that thrives despite the presence of childhood anxiety.

9.1 The Impact of Anxiety on Family

When a child experiences anxiety, its impact ripples through the entire family, influencing sibling relationships, parental roles, and the overall family dynamic. Understanding how anxiety affects family life is a crucial step in providing the necessary support and creating an environment where each family member can thrive.

First and foremost, anxiety can alter the roles and responsibilities of parents and caregivers within the family. Often, one parent may become more heavily involved in helping the anxious child, attending therapy sessions, or managing anxiety-related challenges. This shift in roles can create stress and potential imbalances in the family, as other children may perceive unequal attention or feel their needs are not being met.

Siblings, in particular, can be significantly impacted by a brother or sister's anxiety. They may witness their sibling's struggles, which can evoke feelings of confusion, worry, or guilt. Siblings may also need to adapt to changes in family routines or dynamics due to the anxious child's needs. These adjustments can lead to mixed emotions, including resentment, compassion, or a sense of responsibility. Thus, understanding and addressing the sibling's feelings and concerns is crucial for fostering healthy family relationships.

The overall family environment may become characterized by heightened stress levels and tension, particularly during challenging moments when the anxious child experiences heightened anxiety or panic attacks. These episodes can be emotionally draining for everyone involved, and it's not uncommon for parents and caregivers to experience increased stress and feelings of helplessness as they navigate the complexities of managing their child's anxiety.

In this chapter, we will explore the multifaceted impact of anxiety on families and provide strategies for parents, caregivers, and siblings to navigate these challenges effectively. By fostering open communication, empathy, and resilience within the family unit, it is possible to create a supportive environment where each member can thrive despite the presence of childhood anxiety.

9.1.1 Empathy and Understanding

Empathy and understanding are the cornerstones of maintaining healthy family dynamics when a child in the family is dealing with anxiety. These qualities foster a supportive environment and help family members navigate the complexities of anxiety-related challenges with compassion and patience.

9.1.1.1 The Role of Empathy and Understanding

Empathy and understanding play several vital roles in the family context of childhood anxiety:

1. Validation: They validate the experiences and emotions of the anxious child, letting them know that their feelings are acknowledged and respected.

2. Reducing Stigma: They help reduce the stigma associated with anxiety by normalizing the discussion of emotions and mental health within the family.

3. Strengthening Relationships: Empathy and understanding strengthen sibling bonds, parent-child relationships, and overall family cohesion by fostering open and supportive communication.

9.1.1.2 Strategies for Cultivating Empathy and Understanding

Here are some strategies to cultivate empathy and understanding within the family:

1. Open Communication: Encourage open and non-judgmental communication within the family, where children can express their thoughts, feelings, and concerns.

2. Active Listening: Teach family members, including siblings, to actively listen to each other without interrupting or offering immediate solutions.

3. Educational Resources: Provide age-appropriate educational resources about anxiety for siblings and family members to enhance their understanding of the condition.

4. Share Experiences: Encourage the anxious child to share their experiences, challenges, and triumphs with the family, helping everyone gain insight into their perspective.

5. Family Meetings: Hold regular family meetings to discuss anxiety-related topics and concerns, involving all family members in problem-solving and decision-making.

6. Encourage Questions: Create an environment where family members, especially siblings, feel comfortable asking questions about anxiety and its effects.

7. Empathy Exercises: Practice empathy-building exercises within the family, such as taking turns sharing how different situations make each person feel.

8. Model Empathy: Model empathy and understanding in your own interactions with the anxious child and other family members.

9. Conflict Resolution: Teach conflict resolution skills to help siblings and family members address disagreements and conflicts with empathy.

10. Supportive Language: Encourage the use of supportive and validating language, such as "I understand that this is hard for you" or "I'm here for you."

11. Respect Boundaries: Respect the boundaries of the anxious child, ensuring they feel safe discussing their anxiety but not pressured to share more than they are comfortable with.

Empathy and understanding within the family create a nurturing environment where the anxious child feels valued and supported, and where siblings learn valuable life skills related to compassion and emotional intelligence. By embracing these qualities, families can navigate the challenges of childhood anxiety while strengthening their bonds and resilience as a unit.

9.1.2 Sibling Support

Sibling support is a vital component of family dynamics when a child in the family is dealing with anxiety. Siblings play a unique role in each other's lives, and their support can significantly impact the anxious child's well-being and the overall family environment.

9.1.2.1 The Importance of Sibling Support

Sibling support carries several essential benefits within the family context of childhood anxiety:

1. Emotional Connection: Siblings can provide emotional support and a sense of connection, helping the anxious child feel understood and less isolated.

2. Normalizing Experiences: Siblings who are well-informed about anxiety can help normalize the anxious child's experiences and feelings, reducing stigma.

3. Learning Empathy: Offering support to a sibling with anxiety can teach empathy, patience, and understanding, valuable life skills that benefit all family members.

4. Strengthened Bonds: Sibling support strengthens relationships, fosters a sense of unity, and promotes a supportive family environment.

9.1.2.2 Strategies for Encouraging Sibling Support

Here are strategies to encourage sibling support within the family:

1. Open Communication: Facilitate open conversations between siblings about anxiety. Encourage them to ask questions and share their thoughts and feelings.

2. Educational Resources: Provide age-appropriate educational materials about anxiety to help siblings understand the condition better.

3. Sibling Involvement: Involve siblings in the anxious child's therapy sessions or treatment plan when appropriate, so they feel included and informed.

4. Empathy-Building Activities: Engage in empathy-building activities as a family, such as storytelling or role-playing, to help siblings better understand anxiety.

5. Encourage Patience: Teach siblings the value of patience and the importance of offering emotional support without judgment.

6. Celebrate Achievements: Acknowledge and celebrate the achievements and progress of the anxious child, reinforcing a positive and supportive atmosphere.

7. Sibling Bonding Time: Create opportunities for siblings to spend quality one-on-one time with each other, nurturing their unique bond.

8. Empower Siblings: Encourage siblings to be advocates for the anxious child when appropriate, such as helping them communicate their needs or concerns to parents or teachers.

9. Respect Boundaries: Emphasize the importance of respecting the anxious child's boundaries and ensuring their comfort when discussing anxiety-related topics.

10. Model Support: Model supportive behavior by demonstrating empathy, understanding, and patience in your interactions with the anxious child and their siblings.

Sibling support is a powerful tool in helping children with anxiety navigate their challenges within the family context. By fostering an environment of empathy and understanding among siblings, parents can create a cohesive family unit that stands strong together, supporting each member's unique needs and fostering resilience.

9.2 Family Bonding Activities

In the midst of managing childhood anxiety within the family, it's essential to prioritize bonding activities that promote unity, understanding, and positive relationships among family members. These activities not only create lasting memories but also strengthen the family's resilience and ability to navigate anxiety-related challenges together.

Family bonding activities provide opportunities for open communication, shared experiences, and the development of empathy. They help create a sense of togetherness, reminding each family member that they can rely on one another for support and understanding. Here are a few ideas for family bonding activities in the context of childhood anxiety:

1. Family Game Nights: Regular game nights allow family members to engage in friendly competition, laughter, and shared enjoyment. Board games, card games, or video games can all be suitable options.

2. Nature Adventures: Spend time in nature as a family by going for hikes, picnics, or camping trips. Nature provides a serene backdrop for conversations and relaxation.

3. Art and Creativity: Encourage family members to express themselves through art, whether it's painting, drawing, or crafting. This creative outlet can serve as a valuable means of communication and self-expression.

4. Cooking Together: Collaborate on cooking or baking projects, allowing everyone to contribute to a

delicious meal or dessert. Preparing and enjoying food together can foster a sense of teamwork.

5. Movie or Book Nights: Choose a movie or book to enjoy together as a family. Afterward, discuss the themes and emotions portrayed in the story, creating an opportunity for meaningful conversations.

6. Community Volunteering: Engage in volunteer activities as a family, contributing to your community while reinforcing the values of empathy and altruism.

7. Family Journaling: Create a family journal where each member can write or draw their thoughts, feelings, and experiences. Sharing the journal can facilitate understanding and empathy.

8. Outdoor Sports and Activities: Participate in outdoor sports or activities that cater to everyone's interests, such as biking, playing catch, or flying kites in the park.

9. Family Meetings: Hold regular family meetings to discuss important topics and share experiences. These meetings can encourage open communication and collaborative problem-solving.

10. Family Photo Albums: Review old family photo albums together, reminiscing about past experiences and reinforcing the bonds that have been built over time.

The key to effective family bonding activities is to create an atmosphere of trust and support, where each family member feels valued and heard. By nurturing these connections, families can better navigate the challenges of childhood anxiety as a cohesive unit, building resilience and reinforcing the understanding that they are in it together, every step of the way.

9.2.1 Quality Time Together

Quality time spent together as a family is an essential aspect of fostering strong relationships and resilience, especially when dealing with childhood anxiety. These moments provide opportunities for open communication, emotional connection, and the reinforcement of the family bond.

9.2.1.1 The Significance of Quality Time

Quality time together offers numerous benefits within the family context:

1. Emotional Connection: Spending quality time together strengthens emotional connections among family members, helping them feel closer and more supported.

2. Communication: These moments create a safe space for open and honest communication, allowing family members to share their thoughts, feelings, and concerns.

3. Stress Reduction: Quality time can serve as a reprieve from the stress and anxiety associated with everyday life, offering relaxation and enjoyment.

4. Conflict Resolution: It provides opportunities to address any conflicts or issues that may arise within the family, promoting resolution and understanding.

9.2.1.2 Strategies for Quality Time Together

Here are some strategies for maximizing quality time together as a family:

1. Family Dinners: Make an effort to have regular family dinners where everyone can sit down, share a meal, and engage in conversations about their day.

2. Tech-Free Time: Dedicate tech-free hours or evenings where screens are put away, allowing for uninterrupted family interactions.

3. Family Rituals: Create family rituals, such as a weekly movie night, a designated game night, or a special Sunday morning breakfast tradition.

4. Shared Hobbies: Identify shared hobbies or interests within the family that everyone can participate in, whether it's gardening, hiking, or cooking.

5. Volunteer as a Family: Engage in volunteer activities as a family, giving back to the community while bonding over a shared sense of purpose.

6. Reading Together: Read books together as a family, taking turns or listening to audiobooks during car rides or before bedtime.

7. Family Projects: Undertake family projects or home improvement tasks that require collaboration and teamwork.

8. Vacations and Getaways: Plan occasional family vacations or weekend getaways to create memorable experiences and strengthen family bonds.

9. Family Meetings: Hold family meetings to discuss important topics, share experiences, and make decisions as a unit.

10. Quality Conversations: Encourage quality conversations by actively listening to each other, asking open-ended questions, and fostering an environment of trust.

Quality time together need not be elaborate or expensive; what matters most is the intention behind it. By dedicating time and attention to family connections, parents and caregivers can help their children feel valued and supported in their journey to manage anxiety. These moments of togetherness become a source of strength and resilience for the entire family, reinforcing the understanding that they are there for each other, no matter the challenges they face.

9.2.2 Group Problem-Solving

Group problem-solving is a valuable family activity that not only strengthens family bonds but also equips family members with essential skills for navigating challenges, including childhood anxiety. This collaborative approach encourages open communication, teamwork, and creative thinking while addressing specific issues or concerns within the family.

9.2.2.1 The Power of Group Problem-Solving

Group problem-solving offers several advantages within the family context:

1. Shared Responsibility: It distributes the responsibility of finding solutions among family members, reinforcing the idea that everyone plays a role in overcoming challenges.

2. Open Communication: Group discussions encourage open and honest communication, enabling family members to express their thoughts and feelings.

3. Conflict Resolution: Group problem-solving provides a structured platform for addressing conflicts or concerns within the family, promoting resolution and understanding.

4. Problem-Solving Skills: It teaches valuable problem-solving skills that family members can apply to various aspects of their lives.

9.2.2.2 Strategies for Group Problem-Solving

Here are strategies for effective group problem-solving as a family:

1. Identify the Issue: Begin by clearly identifying the issue or challenge that needs to be addressed. Ensure that everyone understands the problem.

2. Brainstorm Solutions: Encourage family members to brainstorm possible solutions without judgment. Write down all ideas, no matter how unconventional they may seem.

3. Evaluate Solutions: Discuss the pros and cons of each solution. Consider the potential impact on each family member and the family as a whole.

4. Choose a Solution: As a group, decide on the best solution or a combination of solutions. Ensure that everyone agrees and commits to the chosen course of action.

5. Create an Action Plan: Outline the steps needed to implement the chosen solution. Assign responsibilities to family members based on their capabilities and availability.

6. Set Goals: Establish specific, measurable, and achievable goals related to the chosen solution. This helps track progress and success.

7. Review and Adjust: Periodically review the progress made and the effectiveness of the chosen solution. Be open to adjusting the plan if necessary.

8. Celebrate Achievements: Celebrate successes and milestones reached along the way. Acknowledge the efforts and contributions of each family member.

9. Conflict Resolution: If conflicts arise during the problem-solving process, address them calmly and constructively, ensuring that everyone feels heard and respected.

10. Positive Reinforcement: Use positive reinforcement to encourage family members to actively participate and engage in the problem-solving process.

Group problem-solving activities can range from addressing everyday challenges, such as managing household chores, to discussing more complex issues, including how to support a family member with anxiety. By involving the entire family in the process, parents and caregivers can create a sense of unity and shared responsibility, reinforcing the understanding that they are a team, capable of overcoming challenges together.

Chapter 10: Thriving Beyond Anxiety

Introduction

The journey of managing childhood anxiety is not solely about overcoming challenges; it's also about thriving beyond them. In this final chapter, we shift our focus from anxiety management to fostering resilience, self-confidence, and a sense of empowerment in children. It's about helping them embrace life's opportunities, challenges, and adventures with courage and enthusiasm.

Anxiety may remain a part of a child's life, but it doesn't have to define their future. Instead, it can be a catalyst for growth, self-discovery, and building a brighter, more fulfilling path forward. In this chapter, we explore strategies for helping children thrive despite anxiety, emphasizing the importance of resilience, self-esteem, and a positive mindset.

By nurturing these qualities and providing children with the tools they need to manage anxiety effectively, we empower them to not only face their fears but to also chase their dreams and aspirations. It's about encouraging children to believe in themselves, pursue their passions, and build a life filled with joy, purpose, and resilience.

As we embark on this final chapter, let us celebrate the progress made, the challenges overcome, and the potential that lies ahead. Together, we can inspire children to thrive beyond anxiety, nurturing their unique strengths and resilience, and helping them lead fulfilling lives filled with hope and optimism.

10.1 Monitoring Progress

Monitoring progress is a crucial aspect of helping children thrive beyond anxiety. It involves tracking their journey of managing anxiety, celebrating successes, and identifying areas where growth and improvement are possible. By actively monitoring progress, parents, caregivers, and educators can provide children with the encouragement and support they need to continue building resilience and self-confidence.

One of the first steps in monitoring progress is setting clear and achievable goals. These goals should be specific, measurable, and tailored to the child's individual needs and challenges related to anxiety. Whether the goal is to attend a social event without excessive worry or to perform well in school, having a defined target helps both the child and those supporting them track their development.

Regular check-ins and discussions about progress are essential. Engage the child in conversations about their experiences, emotions, and the strategies they've been using to manage anxiety. Encourage them to reflect on their achievements, no matter how small, and acknowledge their efforts. These discussions foster a sense of ownership over their progress and help them recognize their resilience.

Monitoring progress isn't just about assessing the child's anxiety-related goals; it's also about evaluating their overall well-being. Pay attention to changes in their behavior, mood, and physical health. Are they sleeping better? Are they participating in activities they enjoy? Are they showing increased self-esteem? These indicators provide valuable insights into their overall development.

Additionally, consider involving professionals, such as therapists or counselors, in the monitoring process. They can offer expert guidance and objective assessments of the child's progress. Collaborative discussions with these experts can help fine-tune strategies and interventions to better meet the child's needs.

Remember that progress is not always linear. There may be setbacks and challenging moments along the way, and that's perfectly normal. The key is to view these setbacks as opportunities for growth and learning. Encourage the child to approach setbacks with resilience, self-compassion, and a determination to continue their journey towards thriving beyond anxiety.

In the process of monitoring progress, we not only celebrate the milestones achieved but also reinforce the child's belief in their ability to conquer anxiety. By keeping a watchful eye on their development and providing unwavering support, we empower them to build a future filled with confidence, resilience, and endless possibilities.

10.1.1 Keeping a Journal

One effective way to monitor progress in a child's journey to thrive beyond anxiety is by encouraging them to keep a journal. Journaling serves as a valuable tool for self-reflection, tracking emotions, and celebrating achievements. It allows children to gain insight into their experiences, recognize patterns, and set goals for continued growth.

10.1.1.1 The Benefits of Keeping a Journal

Keeping a journal offers several benefits in the context of managing anxiety and fostering resilience:

1. Emotional Awareness: Journaling helps children develop emotional intelligence by identifying and labeling their emotions, which is essential for managing anxiety effectively.

2. Self-Reflection: It provides a space for self-reflection, allowing children to explore the underlying causes of their anxiety and gain clarity on their thought patterns.

3. Goal Setting: Journaling encourages the setting of specific goals related to anxiety management, tracking progress toward those goals, and celebrating milestones.

4. Stress Reduction: Writing down thoughts and emotions can serve as a form of emotional release, reducing stress and promoting mental well-being.

5. Problem-Solving: It supports problem-solving by enabling children to brainstorm potential solutions to anxiety-related challenges.

10.1.1.2 Strategies for Keeping a Journal

Here are strategies to help children keep an effective journal for monitoring their progress:

1. Choose a Journal: Let the child select a journal that resonates with them, whether it's a traditional paper journal or a digital one.

2. Set a Routine: Establish a consistent journaling routine, whether it's daily, weekly, or as needed.

Consistency enhances the journal's effectiveness.

3. Prompts and Questions: Provide prompts or questions to guide journal entries, such as "What made me anxious today?" or "What strategies did I use to manage my anxiety?"

4. Emotion Tracking: Encourage children to record their emotions, including the intensity and duration of anxiety-related feelings.

5. Celebrate Achievements: Create a section in the journal to celebrate achievements and progress. Encourage children to write about their successes, no matter how small.

6. Identify Triggers: Help children identify triggers for their anxiety and explore how these triggers can be managed or avoided.

7. Mindfulness Exercises: Include mindfulness exercises or gratitude journaling to foster a positive mindset and resilience.

8. Reflect on Strategies: Encourage children to reflect on the effectiveness of the strategies they've been using to manage anxiety.

9. Privacy and Safety: Ensure that the journal is a private and safe space for the child to express their thoughts and emotions without judgment.

10. Parental Involvement: If the child is comfortable, allow them to share their journal entries with you, facilitating open conversations and additional support.

Keeping a journal can be a powerful tool in a child's journey to thrive beyond anxiety. It provides them with a sense of control and self-awareness while fostering resilience and emotional growth. By nurturing this practice, parents, caregivers, and educators empower children to navigate their anxiety with insight and confidence, ultimately building a future filled with resilience and emotional well-being.

10.1.2 Tracking Achievements

Monitoring progress in a child's journey to thrive beyond anxiety involves the essential practice of tracking achievements. Recognizing and celebrating accomplishments, no matter how small, can boost a child's self-esteem, motivation, and overall sense of progress. It reinforces the belief that they have the capability to overcome challenges and grow stronger in the face of anxiety.

10.1.2.1 The Significance of Tracking Achievements

Tracking achievements holds several significant advantages:

1. Self-Esteem Boost: Celebrating achievements enhances a child's self-esteem and self-worth, contributing to their overall well-being.

2. Motivation: It motivates children to continue their efforts in managing anxiety and working towards their goals.

3. Positive Reinforcement: Recognizing achievements reinforces the effectiveness of anxiety management strategies and encourages their continued use.

4. Emotional Resilience: It helps build emotional resilience by focusing on strengths and successes, rather than dwelling on challenges.

10.1.2.2 Strategies for Tracking Achievements

Here are strategies for effectively tracking achievements in a child's journey to thrive beyond anxiety:

1. Define Clear Goals: Ensure that the child has specific, measurable goals related to anxiety management. These goals provide a clear path for tracking progress.

2. Create an Achievement Journal: Designate a journal or chart specifically for tracking achievements related to anxiety management.

3. Regular Check-Ins: Schedule regular check-in sessions with the child to discuss their progress and celebrate achievements together.

4. Positive Reinforcement: Use positive reinforcement, such as praise and rewards, to acknowledge achievements and motivate continued effort.

5. Record Achievements: Encourage the child to record their achievements in their journal, noting what they accomplished, how it made them feel, and any strategies they used.

6. Milestone Celebrations: Celebrate significant milestones along the journey, whether it's completing a challenging task, facing a fear, or consistently practicing anxiety management techniques.

7. Family Involvement: Involve the family in celebrating achievements, fostering a supportive environment where everyone acknowledges and values progress.

8. Visual Aids: Create visual aids, such as progress charts or vision boards, to visualize the child's goals and achievements.

9. Reflect on Growth: Prompt the child to reflect on their personal growth and resilience as they achieve their anxiety-related goals.

10. Set New Goals: After achieving a goal, work with the child to set new ones, ensuring that the journey of progress continues.

Tracking achievements is not only a means of celebrating past successes but also a way to inspire confidence in facing future challenges. It reinforces the idea that managing anxiety is an ongoing journey filled with opportunities for growth and personal development. By tracking achievements together, parents, caregivers, and educators can play a pivotal role in helping children thrive beyond anxiety, cultivating a sense of accomplishment and empowerment that will serve them well throughout their lives.

10.2 Celebrating Successes

Celebrating successes is a fundamental aspect of helping children thrive beyond anxiety. It is a way of recognizing and reinforcing their achievements, no matter how small or large, and nurturing a sense of pride and self-worth. Celebrations not only boost a child's confidence but also encourage them to persist in their efforts to manage anxiety effectively.

One of the key elements of celebrating successes is acknowledging that progress is not solely measured by the absence of anxiety but by the steps taken to confront and overcome it. Successes can take various forms, from facing a fear or participating in a social event to effectively using anxiety management techniques. By acknowledging these achievements, parents, caregivers, and educators validate the child's resilience and determination.

Celebrations serve as powerful positive reinforcement. They send the message that the child's efforts and hard work are noticed and appreciated. This reinforcement can motivate the child to continue using effective anxiety management strategies, creating a cycle of growth and progress.

It's essential to customize celebrations to the child's preferences and interests. Some children may appreciate verbal praise, while others might prefer tangible rewards or special experiences. The key is to make celebrations meaningful and tailored to the individual, ensuring that they feel genuinely valued and encouraged.

Moreover, celebrations don't only happen at the end of the journey; they can occur at various milestones along the way. By acknowledging each step of progress, parents, caregivers, and educators create a positive and motivating atmosphere that reinforces the child's belief in their ability to thrive beyond anxiety.

Ultimately, celebrating successes is about fostering resilience, self-esteem, and a positive mindset in children. It teaches them that even in the face of anxiety, they can achieve and overcome. These celebrations serve as a reminder that they have the strength to confront challenges, chase their dreams, and build a future filled with hope and optimism.

10.2.1 Gradual Steps Toward Independence

One of the most significant successes a child can achieve in their journey to thrive beyond anxiety is the development of independence. While anxiety can create a sense of dependency, fostering independence allows children to build resilience, self-confidence, and a belief in their ability to navigate life's challenges.

10.2.1.1 The Importance of Gradual Independence

Gradual steps toward independence hold several significant benefits:

1. Resilience Building: Encouraging independence fosters resilience by teaching children to face and overcome obstacles on their own.

2. Self-Confidence: As children accomplish tasks independently, their self-confidence grows, bolstering their belief in their capabilities.

3. Problem-Solving Skills: Independence promotes problem-solving skills, as children learn to make decisions and manage challenges autonomously.

4. Empowerment: It empowers children to take ownership of their lives, make choices, and set goals for their future.

10.2.1.2 Strategies for Fostering Gradual Independence

Here are strategies to help children take gradual steps toward independence:

1. Identify Age-Appropriate Tasks: Determine tasks or responsibilities that are suitable for the child's age and maturity level.

2. Set Clear Expectations: Clearly communicate expectations for each task, emphasizing the child's responsibility and autonomy.

3. Provide Guidance: Offer guidance and support as needed, ensuring that the child feels confident in completing the task independently.

4. Offer Choices: Give children opportunities to make choices within boundaries, allowing them to practice decision-making.

5. Encourage Problem-Solving: Prompt children to think critically and problem-solve when challenges arise during a task.

6. Celebrate Achievements: Celebrate each successful completion of a task or step toward independence, reinforcing their sense of accomplishment.

7. Gradual Progression: Gradually increase the complexity of tasks and responsibilities as the child demonstrates readiness and confidence.

8. Open Communication: Maintain open communication, allowing the child to express their feelings, concerns, and preferences throughout the process.

9. Reinforce Resilience: When setbacks occur, emphasize the importance of resilience and the opportunity to learn from challenges.

10. Support from Afar: As the child becomes more independent, offer support from a distance, ensuring they know you are available if needed.

Fostering gradual independence is a key success in a child's journey to thrive beyond anxiety. It equips them with essential life skills, empowers them to make choices, and instills the belief that they are capable of managing challenges independently. Through this process, children develop the self-confidence and resilience needed to embrace life's opportunities and create a future filled with confidence and autonomy.

10.2.2 Planning for the Future

Planning for the future is a significant milestone in helping children thrive beyond anxiety. It involves fostering a forward-thinking mindset and equipping children with the skills and confidence to envision and pursue their goals and aspirations. By instilling a sense of purpose and direction, parents, caregivers, and educators empower children to build a future filled with hope and optimism.

10.2.2.1 The Significance of Future Planning

Planning for the future carries several vital benefits:

1. Goal Setting: It encourages children to set meaningful goals and work towards achieving them, providing a sense of purpose and motivation.

2. Long-Term Vision: Future planning helps children develop a long-term vision for their lives, fostering resilience and adaptability.

3. Empowerment: It empowers children to take control of their destiny and make choices that align with their values and aspirations.

4. Decision-Making Skills: Future planning hones decision-making skills, as children learn to weigh options and consider the potential consequences of their choices.

10.2.2.2 Strategies for Future Planning

Here are strategies to help children plan for their future:

1. Encourage Dreaming: Prompt children to dream and imagine their ideal future, emphasizing that anything is possible with determination and effort.

2. Set Achievable Goals: Help children set achievable short-term and long-term goals, ensuring they are specific, measurable, and aligned with their interests and values.

3. Career Exploration: Introduce children to various careers and fields of interest, fostering a sense of curiosity and exploration.

4. Education and Skill Development: Discuss the importance of education and skill development as tools for achieving their goals.

5. Time Management: Teach time management skills to help children balance their academic, extracurricular, and personal pursuits.

6. Problem-Solving: Encourage problem-solving by discussing potential obstacles and challenges they might encounter on their path to their goals.

7. Supportive Environment: Create a supportive environment where children feel comfortable sharing their aspirations and discussing their future plans.

8. Celebrate Milestones: Celebrate milestones and achievements related to future planning, reinforcing

their belief in their ability to shape their destiny.

9. Model Planning: Model future planning by sharing your own goals and aspirations, demonstrating the value of setting and working towards objectives.

10. Emphasize Resilience: Remind children that setbacks and challenges are a natural part of pursuing one's dreams and that resilience is key to overcoming them.

Planning for the future instills hope and purpose in children's lives. It encourages them to envision a future where anxiety does not define their potential or limit their opportunities. By nurturing their ability to plan and pursue their goals, parents, caregivers, and educators provide children with the tools to build a future filled with confidence, optimism, and the belief that they can thrive beyond anxiety.

Chapter 11: Resources for Parents and Caregivers

Introduction

The journey of supporting a child through anxiety can be both rewarding and challenging. As parents and caregivers, your unwavering love and dedication play a pivotal role in helping children thrive beyond anxiety. However, it's essential to recognize that you are not alone on this journey. This chapter is dedicated to providing you with a comprehensive list of resources, tools, and support networks to assist you in guiding your child through anxiety and building a resilient, thriving future together.

Navigating childhood anxiety requires a multifaceted approach that includes education, professional guidance, and a support system. In this chapter, we aim to equip you with a wide range of resources that encompass all aspects of your child's well-being, from understanding anxiety to seeking professional help, creating a supportive environment, and fostering resilience.

Each resource listed is carefully selected to provide you with valuable information, strategies, and assistance tailored to your unique needs as a parent or caregiver. Whether you're seeking expert advice, looking for educational materials, or exploring support networks, you'll find a wealth of resources to help you effectively support your child in managing anxiety and thriving beyond it.

As you continue on your journey, remember that seeking help and utilizing available resources is a sign of strength and dedication to your child's well-being. Together, we can provide the support and guidance your child needs to overcome anxiety and build a future filled with confidence, resilience, and endless possibilities.

11.1 Books and Websites

Books and websites are valuable resources for parents and caregivers seeking information, guidance, and strategies to support their children in managing anxiety. Whether you prefer reading comprehensive guides or accessing up-to-date information online, these resources offer a wealth of knowledge and practical advice to help you navigate the challenges of childhood anxiety.

Books:

1. "The Anxiety and Phobia Workbook" by Edmund J. Bourne: This widely acclaimed book provides practical exercises, techniques, and strategies for managing anxiety, making it a valuable resource for

both parents and children.

2. "Freeing Your Child from Anxiety" by Tamar E. Chansky: Dr. Chansky offers insights into understanding childhood anxiety and provides parents with effective tools to help their children overcome anxiety-related challenges.

3. "The Opposite of Worry" by Lawrence J. Cohen: This book focuses on building resilience in children and offers strategies to reduce anxiety and promote emotional well-being.

4. "Helping Your Anxious Child" by Ronald M. Rapee, Ann Wignall, Susan Spence, and Heidi Lyneham: Written by leading experts, this book provides practical guidance on understanding and managing childhood anxiety.

Websites:

1. Anxiety and Depression Association of America (ADAA) - Child and Adolescent Anxiety: ADAA offers a dedicated section with articles, resources, and expert advice on childhood anxiety.

2. Child Mind Institute: This organization provides a wealth of information and resources related to children's mental health, including anxiety disorders.

3. National Institute of Mental Health (NIMH) - Child and Adolescent Mental Health: NIMH offers valuable insights into the latest research and treatment options for children with mental health conditions, including anxiety.

4. Childhood Anxiety Network: This online community provides support, articles, and resources for parents dealing with childhood anxiety.

5. Understood.org: Focused on children with learning and attention issues, this website offers resources and expert advice for parents navigating various challenges, including anxiety.

These books and websites serve as valuable sources of information, offering practical tips, expert guidance, and the latest research on childhood anxiety. They can help parents and caregivers gain a deeper understanding of anxiety, equip them with effective strategies for supporting their children, and connect them with supportive communities and networks. By utilizing these resources, you can empower yourself to provide the best possible support for your child as they navigate their journey toward thriving beyond anxiety.

11.2 Support Groups and Counseling Services

Support groups and counseling services play a crucial role in providing parents and caregivers with the guidance, empathy, and professional assistance needed to navigate childhood anxiety effectively. These resources offer a safe space to share experiences, gain insights, and access expert support, helping you and your child cope with anxiety and work towards a brighter future.

Support Groups:

1. Local Parent Support Groups: Many local organizations and mental health centers host support groups for parents and caregivers of children with anxiety. These groups offer a supportive community

where you can share experiences, exchange coping strategies, and find solace in knowing you're not alone on this journey.

2. Online Support Communities: Numerous online forums and social media groups are dedicated to parents and caregivers dealing with childhood anxiety. These virtual communities allow you to connect with others facing similar challenges, seek advice, and provide and receive support from the comfort of your home.

3. School-Based Support: Some schools and educational institutions offer parent support groups as part of their efforts to address childhood anxiety. These groups often involve discussions on school-related challenges and solutions.

Counseling Services:

1. Individual Therapy: Seeking therapy for yourself can be invaluable in managing the stress and emotions that come with supporting a child with anxiety. A trained therapist can offer guidance and teach coping strategies tailored to your specific situation.

2. Family Therapy: Family therapy sessions can help improve communication and relationships within the family unit, addressing any dynamics that may contribute to a child's anxiety.

3. Child and Adolescent Counseling: For your child, seeking the expertise of a child psychologist or counselor can provide them with tools to manage anxiety, explore its root causes, and develop coping mechanisms.

4. Parent-Child Counseling: This form of counseling involves both you and your child, allowing you to work together to address anxiety-related challenges as a team.

5. Online Counseling Services: Many therapists offer online counseling sessions, providing convenient access to professional help from the comfort of your home.

Remember that seeking support through these channels is a proactive step towards better understanding and managing childhood anxiety. Whether you choose to participate in a support group, seek individual counseling, or explore family therapy, these resources can offer valuable insights, emotional support, and practical strategies to help both you and your child thrive beyond anxiety.

11.3 Advocacy and Awareness Organizations

Advocacy and awareness organizations are instrumental in the fight against childhood anxiety. These organizations work tirelessly to raise awareness, reduce stigma, and drive positive change in the field of mental health. As a parent or caregiver, engaging with these organizations can provide you with a wealth of information, support, and opportunities to advocate for better mental health care for your child and others.

National Alliance on Mental Illness (NAMI): NAMI is a prominent advocacy organization that offers resources, support, and educational programs for individuals and families affected by mental health conditions, including anxiety disorders in children. They advocate for improved mental health policies and access to quality care.

Anxiety and Depression Association of America (ADAA): ADAA is dedicated to promoting the prevention, treatment, and cure of anxiety and depression. They offer resources, webinars, and expert advice on anxiety disorders in children and work to reduce stigma surrounding mental health.

Child Mind Institute: This organization is committed to transforming the lives of children struggling with mental health and learning disorders. They provide comprehensive resources, offer telehealth services, and conduct research to improve the understanding and treatment of childhood anxiety.

The Trevor Project: While primarily focused on LGBTQ+ youth, The Trevor Project provides resources for parents and caregivers seeking to support children and adolescents dealing with anxiety and other mental health challenges.

National Institute of Mental Health (NIMH): NIMH conducts research on mental health conditions, including childhood anxiety, and provides valuable information and resources for families. They aim to advance our understanding of mental health disorders and improve treatment options.

Local and Regional Mental Health Organizations: Depending on your location, there may be local or regional mental health advocacy organizations that offer support, educational events, and resources tailored to your specific community's needs.

Engaging with advocacy and awareness organizations can empower you as a parent or caregiver to become an advocate for your child and others facing childhood anxiety. These organizations provide access to educational materials, research updates, policy initiatives, and opportunities to connect with a supportive community of individuals who share your concerns and goals. By joining forces with these organizations, you can contribute to the collective effort to improve mental health care, reduce stigma, and ensure a brighter future for children living with anxiety.

Chapter 12: Conclusion

The journey of helping children thrive beyond anxiety is one of courage, resilience, and unwavering love. Throughout this book, we've explored the complexities of childhood anxiety and provided you with a comprehensive guide to understand, support, and empower your child to overcome these challenges.

In the midst of this journey, you've learned that anxiety is not an insurmountable obstacle but a hurdle that, with the right strategies and support, your child can learn to overcome. It's important to remember that progress may not always be linear, and setbacks are a natural part of growth. As parents and caregivers, your role is not to eliminate anxiety entirely but to equip your child with the tools to manage it effectively.

Here are some key takeaways from our journey together:

1. Understanding Anxiety: You've gained insights into the different types of anxiety disorders, recognizing anxiety's signs, and understanding its impact on your child's life.

2. Early Intervention: The importance of early intervention in addressing childhood anxiety cannot be overstated. Timely support and professional help can make a significant difference in your child's well-being.

3. Building a Supportive Environment: Creating a safe, nurturing, and empathetic environment at home and school is essential. Active listening, setting realistic expectations, and encouraging self-care are crucial components of this support.

4. Coping Strategies: We explored various coping strategies, including mindfulness techniques, cognitive-behavioral approaches, and healthy lifestyle habits that can empower your child to manage anxiety effectively.

5. Thriving Beyond Anxiety: Your child's journey isn't just about managing anxiety; it's about thriving beyond it. By fostering resilience, self-esteem, independence, and future planning, you help them build a future filled with hope and optimism.

6. Resources and Support: We've provided you with a wealth of resources, from books and websites to support groups, counseling services, and advocacy organizations. These resources are invaluable in your ongoing journey.

Remember that you are not alone in this journey. Seek support when needed, both for yourself and your child. Embrace the small victories and celebrate successes together. Continue to communicate openly and foster a loving, supportive atmosphere that encourages your child to grow, learn, and thrive.

As we conclude this book, we want to leave you with a message of hope. Your child has immense potential, and anxiety does not define their future. With your guidance, love, and the tools you've acquired, they can face challenges with courage, build resilience, and embrace a future filled with endless possibilities.

The journey may have its ups and downs, but it is a journey worth taking. Your child's well-being is worth every effort, every setback, and every triumph. Keep moving forward, believing in your child's strength, and nurturing their ability to thrive beyond anxiety. Together, you can build a future filled with confidence, resilience, and a deep sense of joy and fulfillment.

12.1 The Journey Ahead

As we close this book, it's essential to acknowledge that the journey of helping your child thrive beyond anxiety is ongoing. While we've covered a wide range of strategies, insights, and resources, the path forward will be uniquely shaped by your child's needs, strengths, and individual journey. Here are some key considerations for the journey ahead:

1. Continued Growth: Recognize that growth is a continuous process. Your child may face new challenges and anxieties as they progress through different stages of life. Be prepared to adapt and learn alongside them.

2. Open Communication: Keep the lines of communication open with your child. Encourage them to share their thoughts, feelings, and concerns with you. This open dialogue will help you stay attuned to their needs.

3. Professional Support: If you haven't already, consider seeking professional help if your child's anxiety persists or worsens. Therapists, counselors, and mental health professionals can provide specialized guidance tailored to your child's situation.

4. Empower Independence: Continue to foster your child's independence. Encourage them to apply the coping strategies and life skills they've learned to face anxiety and life's challenges with confidence.

5. Celebrate Successes: Keep celebrating your child's successes, no matter how small. These celebrations reinforce their belief in their ability to manage anxiety and build resilience.

6. Self-Care: Remember that taking care of yourself is essential. Caring for a child with anxiety can be emotionally taxing, so prioritize self-care to ensure you have the energy and resilience needed to support your child effectively.

7. Advocacy: Consider becoming an advocate for mental health awareness and support. Your experiences and insights can contribute to reducing the stigma surrounding anxiety and improving resources and services for children.

8. Connection: Stay connected with the supportive community you've built, whether it's through support groups, counseling, or online networks. These connections can offer ongoing guidance and understanding.

9. Adaptability: Be adaptable in your approach. What works for your child may change over time, so be open to exploring new strategies and seeking fresh insights.

10. Hope: Finally, hold onto hope. Your child has the potential to not only manage anxiety but to flourish in life. With your love, support, and the knowledge you've gained, you are well-equipped to continue guiding them on this journey.

The journey ahead may present its share of challenges, but it also holds countless opportunities for growth, resilience, and joy. Embrace each moment, cherish your child's progress, and keep nurturing their ability to thrive beyond anxiety. Your dedication and love are powerful forces, capable of shaping a future filled with optimism and endless possibilities.

12.2 Empowering Kids for Life

Empowering your child to thrive beyond anxiety is about more than just managing their current challenges; it's about equipping them with life skills, resilience, and a sense of self-worth that will serve them well throughout their lives. Here are some key ways to empower your child for life:

1. Self-Awareness: Encourage your child to develop self-awareness. Help them understand their strengths, weaknesses, and emotions. When they can identify and express their feelings, they're better equipped to manage them.

2. Emotional Intelligence: Teach your child emotional intelligence. Help them recognize emotions in themselves and others, and provide tools for regulating and expressing those emotions in healthy ways.

3. Problem-Solving Skills: Foster problem-solving skills by involving your child in decision-making processes. Encourage them to brainstorm solutions to challenges and evaluate the pros and cons of different options.

4. Resilience: Emphasize the importance of resilience. Let your child know that setbacks and failures are natural parts of life. Teach them to bounce back, learn from their experiences, and keep moving

forward.

5. Effective Communication: Teach effective communication skills. Encourage your child to express themselves assertively and to listen actively to others. These skills are valuable in personal relationships, academics, and future careers.

6. Goal Setting: Continue setting achievable goals with your child. This practice helps them develop a sense of purpose and motivation. Celebrate their achievements and use setbacks as opportunities for growth.

7. Time Management: Introduce time management skills early on. Teach your child how to prioritize tasks, set schedules, and allocate time for responsibilities and leisure activities.

8. Healthy Lifestyle: Continue emphasizing the importance of a healthy lifestyle. Encourage regular physical activity, a balanced diet, and adequate sleep. These habits contribute to overall well-being.

9. Independence: Encourage your child's independence. Allow them to make age-appropriate decisions and learn from their experiences, even if it means making mistakes along the way.

10. Curiosity and Lifelong Learning: Foster a love of learning and curiosity in your child. Encourage them to explore new interests, ask questions, and seek knowledge throughout their lives.

11. Adaptability: Teach adaptability as a valuable skill. Life is full of unexpected changes, and the ability to adapt and stay flexible is a crucial life skill.

12. Empathy and Compassion: Instill empathy and compassion in your child. Help them understand the perspectives and feelings of others. These qualities are fundamental for building meaningful relationships.

By focusing on these life skills and values, you empower your child to not only manage anxiety but also lead a fulfilling and successful life. Remember that your role as a parent or caregiver is not only to provide support but also to guide your child toward becoming a confident, resilient, and compassionate individual who is ready to embrace life's opportunities and challenges with open arms.